7 HABITS *of* HEALTHY AGING

How To Control Aging & Prolong Vitality

*A Step-By-Step Program
To Add Years To Your Life and Life To Your Years*

DR. DONALD L. HAYES

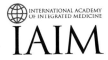

International Academy of Integrated Medicine

Innovative Practice Solutions, Inc.
100 Avenida La Pata
San Clemente, CA 92673
949-369-5980
Fax: 949-369-5981
(800-761-0011)

First Edition 2001

ActualAge™ is patent pending and a registered trademark of Innovative Practice Solutions, Inc.

7 Habits of Healthy Aging is not intended as medical advice. Its intent is solely informational and educational. Please consult a medical or health professional should the need for one be indicated.

Library of Congress Cataloging-in-Publication Data

Hayes, Donald L.
7 Habits of Healthy Aging: How To Control Aging & Prolong Vitality
A Step-By-Step Program To Add Years To Your Life And Life To Your Years/Dr. Donald L. Hayes – 1st ed.

1. Longevity.   2. Aging   3. Health   I. Donald L. Hayes   II. Title

Printed and bound in the United States of America

ISBN: 0-9712993-0-7

Acknowledgements

It's impossible to thank all the people who have helped me in so many ways while on the path to writing this book, but I'll try. I must first of all acknowledge my brother John Hayes whose love and support has helped me all my life. Thanks, John, for showing me what courage really is.

I also want to thank Jeff Katke. Jeff has been a pillar of strength, a breath of fresh air, an innovator of ideas, a supporter of concepts and has challenged me to always do my best. Through it all, he has remained a dear friend. I must thank the entire Katke family, Jim, Marie, Mike, Chris, Tim and Julie, wow, what a beautiful group of human beings. I also want to thank all the Metagenics Distributors worldwide as well as the hundreds of sales managers, representatives, office staff and stockroom personnel.

I truly want to thank Jeff Bland, and the entire team at Healthcom and The Institute For Functional Medicine, for their steadfast dedication to the field of functional medicine. Knowing all of you has changed my life forever.

Thanks to John Burke and the team at Outlook International for their dedication and ongoing support.

I want to give special thanks to Dina Snow of Azteca Design. Her talent helped us create the graphic designs and layouts for the entire program.

And last, I want to thank all the thousands of patients that I had the pleasure of working with over nearly 20 years of clinical practice. It is for many thousands more just like you that I hope the information in this book will help to serve.

Donald L. Hayes, D.C.
San Clemente, CA

Dedication

I dedicate this book to the three women in my life that have taught me how to live, love and laugh. They are first of all my dear mother, Hazel Hayes, who would have been 85 years old the day I finished this book. Without her, I wouldn't have been here to undertake this very important task. She always instructed me to "hang in there," which was much needed advice on those late nights. Thanks, Mom, miss you.

The next is my beautiful daughter, Courtney Hayes, whose smiles and precious laughter motivate me to maintain my own health and vitality so that I may remain on this planet as long as possible to spend time "just hanging" with her. Thanks, "Punky."

And finally to my lovely wife, Deonn Hayes, who is as responsible for this book as I am. Deonn, you are truly the wind beneath my wings, the person who makes me laugh, and feel alive! Thanks, "soulmate," I'll always love and cherish you!

An Important Note:

The information in this book is for educational purposes only. It is not intended, and should not be considered, as a replacement for consultation, diagnosis or treatment by a duly licensed health practitioner.

Contents Page

Introduction

WELCOME TO THE HEALTHY AGING PROGRAM

It doesn't matter who you are or what you do, you absolutely, positively have the power to change your life.

Imagine waking up in the morning feeling great! You bounce out of bed with the kind of energy that will take you from morning to evening. You have the confidence to finally get to all of those things you have been putting off. You are gaining control of your health and control of your life.

That is what the Healthy Aging Program is all about. It doesn't matter if you are old or young, a man or a woman, in great shape or have never exercised before, this program can help you increase your energy, improve your shape and maximize your overall well-being.

So if you are willing to make the commitment and take the next step by following the recommendations outlined in this book, you will make a gigantic leap towards gaining control of not only how you look and feel, but every aspect of your life.

The process begins the minute you turn the page…

UNLOCK THE SECRETS TO HEALTHY AGING

Forget your chronological age from now on; your age in years has little to do with how old you are biologically and how old you feel. Think about your body's age only in terms of the biomarkers of aging that can be measured, monitored, and improved through the implementation of the 7 Habits of Healthy Aging. This book will provide a step-by-step guide on what to do.

HORMONE BALANCE IS THE KEY TO HEALTHY AGING

Hormones are chemical communicators produced in the body that direct the body to break down and create new cells. When a hormone becomes imbalanced, it affects other processes in the body that may lead to a decline in overall hormone levels. If this condition breaks down more cells than it builds up, the end result is aging. This process has been referred to as "sarcopenia." Sarcopenia, by definition, is an overall weakening of the body caused by a change in body composition with a loss of muscle mass.

A recognized expert in human nutrition and functional medicine, Jeffrey S. Bland, Ph.D., president of The Institute for Functional Medicine and author of *Genetic Nutritioneering*, states, "When insulin levels in the blood become very high, they influence gene expression, altering cellular effects and promoting accelerated aging." He adds, "Recent discoveries may lead to a greater understanding of how the control of blood sugar through diet and lifestyle may help reduce biological aging."

The 7 Habits of Healthy Aging Program is designed to balance the body's insulin levels and other hormones through balanced eating, improved eating frequency, exercise, stimulant and stress reduction, and natural supplements. The end result is a program that not only helps control aging, but also helps prevent chronic disease and maximize your health potential.

3 STAGES OF ACCELERATED AGING (SEE FIGURE 1, PAGE 16)

This chart provides a visual overview on how accelerated aging occurs in three distinct stages.

STAGE #1 HIGH-INSULIN LIFESTYLE HABITS

One of the main causes of accelerated aging is high levels of blood insulin due to poor lifestyle habits. High-insulin lifestyle habits include imbalanced eating of the three major macronutrients (carbohydrates, fats and proteins), skipping meals, lack of exercise, use of stimulants like sugar, caffeine, alcohol and tobacco, poor stress management, lack of proper micronutrients (vitamins and minerals), and poor hormone balance.

STAGE #2 HYPERINSULINEMIA

The cells of our body need blood-sugar (glucose) for energy. However, glucose cannot simply flow into the cells from the bloodstream; it must be guided in by insulin, a protein secreted by the pancreas. Hyperinsulinemia is an excess circulation of insulin through the body due to an excess of sugar in the diet, typically caused by following a high-insulin lifestyle. By the time a patient is diagnosed with a high blood-sugar (glucose) level, he or she has been living a high-insulin lifestyle and on the accelerated aging path for some time.

STAGE #3 INSULIN RESISTANCE

Many years of following a high-insulin lifestyle, like eating high carbohydrate, imbalanced meals, causes the body to accumulate excessive sugar. After years of this type of pattern, the cells of the body become saturated with sugar and cannot admit any more sugar (glucose) molecules through the cell membranes. The cells of the body protect themselves from this sugar overload by reducing the number of insulin receptors on the cells, so less sugar is absorbed. This is insulin resistance. In an attempt to overcome the resistance, the pancreas goes into overtime and secretes even more insulin to override the resistance, worsening the condition of hyperinsulinemia.

SYNDROME X

Insulin resistance is associated with Syndrome X, a condition characterized by elevated insulin levels in the blood and a variety of additional manifestations including: excess blood fat, increased body fat, increased waist-to-hip ratio and high blood pressure. Several studies have made it clear that insulin resistance and compensatory hyperinsulinemia, the hallmarks of Syndrome X, tend to raise blood pressure. In fact, the study showed that half of all patients with high blood pressure are insulin resistant, and have one or more components of Syndrome X.

SYNDROME X VERSUS TYPE II DIABETES

Insulin is involved with both Syndrome X and Type II diabetes. In Type II diabetes, insulin is not working as effectively as it should be. When sugar (glucose) from food eaten enters the bloodstream, the pancreas does its best to secrete enough insulin to overcome the insulin resistance and deliver the glucose into the cells. If the pancreas cannot keep up the effort, the amount of sugar in the blood will continue to rise until there's so much, it begins entering the cells by sheer force. When this happens, a person has Type II diabetes. All that excess glucose in the bloodstream causes damage that can lead to blindness, kidney failure and other problems.

Something similar happens with Syndrome X: the insulin pumped out by the pancreas isn't able to deliver glucose into the cells properly. But the difference with Syndrome X is the pancreas shifts into overdrive, putting out more and more insulin until all the glucose has been delivered into the cells.

The difference between Syndrome X and Type II diabetes is that people with Syndrome X can continue pumping out the high amounts of insulin needed to use glucose normally, while those with Type II diabetes cannot. Being able to produce enough insulin to overcome insulin resistance keeps your blood sugar from going too high, so you don't suffer from Type II diabetes and its many serious problems. Unfortunately, a person is left with a very high level of insulin in their bloodstream, amounts that can lead to the many risk factors for Syndrome X and heart disease. And, to make matters worse, the ability of the pancreas to produce insulin may lessen over time, adding Type II diabetes to the list of possible future health risks.

RISK FACTORS FOR DISEASES OF AGING

The various manifestations of Syndrome X are also the major risk factors for diseases of aging such as heart disease, stroke, Type II diabetes and cancer. Although being insulin resistant does not, by itself, mean that you will develop Syndrome X, it is clear that the combination of insulin resistance and compensatory hyperinsulinemia increases your risk of developing the disease.

YOUR BODY'S HORMONES ARE INTERRELATED

The human body is interconnected with various systems and mechanisms, not only the obvious systems of bones and muscles, but also systems of hormones and other chemical communicators. Because of this interconnectedness, following a few key lifestyle habits that help balance out one or two of the major hormones will help the body in its attempt to balance out the others. One of the most important hormones to balance in the body is insulin.

Research has demonstrated that the hormone insulin does more than simply control the level of sugar in the blood. It is a hormone that can indirectly influence a variety of other hormones and metabolic functions, including the way the body utilizes calories for energy or deposits them as fat.

Everything you put into your mouth is going to affect insulin in some way. When insulin levels are kept high too long, you end up with a physiology that promotes inflammation, osteoarthritis, cholesterol abnormalities, coronary artery disease, osteoporosis, high blood pressure, stroke, Type II diabetes, loss of muscle mass and accumulation of excess body fat. Prolonged high-insulin levels set off a multitude of chain reactions that disrupt all other hormones and biochemical reactions at the cellular level. This chronic situation leads to accelerated aging.

The question to ask yourself is, "How do you feel?" Do you feel vital and young, or burned out and exhausted? If you're sick and tired of being sick and tired, ask yourself questions about your lifestyle. Are you living a healthy life, or are you eating unbalanced meals, skipping meals, and using stimulants like sugar, alcohol, soda, caffeine and tobacco regularly? Are you leading a stressful life, forgetting to exercise daily, and not taking proper supplements?

7 HABITS OF HEALTHY AGING (SEE FIGURE 2, PAGE 17)
This chart provides a visual overview of how you can control the aging process and increase your vitality regardless of your age.

The answer to health is balance. Balance can only be achieved by following the proper lifestyle habits that promote it on a daily basis. The 7 Habits of Healthy Aging outlined in this book promote insulin balance and help you increase vitality.

On the pages that follow is a step-by-step program to help control aging and prolong vitality. If you're following the information in this book as part of a program in concert with your healthcare provider, be sure to adhere to his or her advice at all times. If you are using this information without the advice of your doctor, be aware that professional support is usually crucial for success. Under no condition should you start an aggressive diet or exercise program without first consulting your primary healthcare provider.

Good luck and good health!

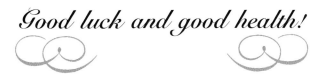

3 STAGES OF ACCELERATED AGING

STAGE #1
HIGH-INSULIN LIFESTYLE HABITS

- Poorly balanced, high carbohydrate meals
- Skipping meals and irregular eating habits
- Lack of a proper exercise program
- Use of stimulants, such as sugar, soda, caffeine
- Lack of stress management
- Micronutrient imbalance
- Hormone imbalances

STAGE #2
HYPERINSULINEMIA

Hyperinsulinemia is an excess circulation of insulin
through the body, typically due to an excess of sugar in the diet.

STAGE #3
INSULIN RESISTANCE - SYNDROME X

Insulin resistance occurs to protect the body from sugar
overload by shutting down insulin receptor sites on the
cells. Insulin resistance is associated with Syndrome X,
a condition closely linked to coronary heart disease.
Insulin resistance triggers the release of even more insulin,
leading to more hyperinsulinemia, a vicious cycle.

RISK FACTORS FOR
DISEASES OF AGING

- High blood pressure
- Abnormal cholesterol metabolism
- High triglyceride levels
- High insulin levels
- Increased body fat
- Increased waist-to-hip ratio
- Decreased muscle mass
- Decreased strength

DISEASES OF AGING

- Heart disease
- Stroke
- Type II diabetes
- Cancer

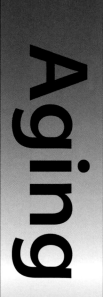

FIGURE 1

7 HABITS OF HEALTHY AGING

HABIT #7 - HORMONE BALANCE

Hormones in the body work together. Just as it's not healthy to have high or low thyroid levels, it's not healthy to have high or low insulin levels. Normal hormone levels indicate balance and help to increase overall vitality.

HABIT #6 - SUPPLEMENT BALANCE

Micronutrient imbalance is an independent risk factor for developing Syndrome X.

HABIT #5 - STRESS MANAGEMENT

For optimum health, regular stress management programs help keep insulin and other hormone levels balanced, improving vitality.

HABIT #4 - REDUCE STIMULANT USE

Regular use of stimulants raises insulin levels and reduces vitality.

HABIT #3 - REGULAR EXERCISE

A regular program of aerobic resistance and flexibility exercises has been shown to reduce insulin levels and reverse insulin sensitivity, that will increase vitality.

HABIT #2 - EATING FREQUENCY

Skipping meals or irregular eating habits increase insulin levels, which decreases vitality.

HABIT #1 - BALANCED EATING

A balanced meal is a meal that has all three of the major macronutrients present: carbohydrates, fats and protein.

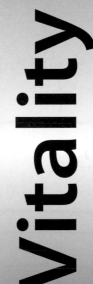

Health

Vitality

FIGURE 2

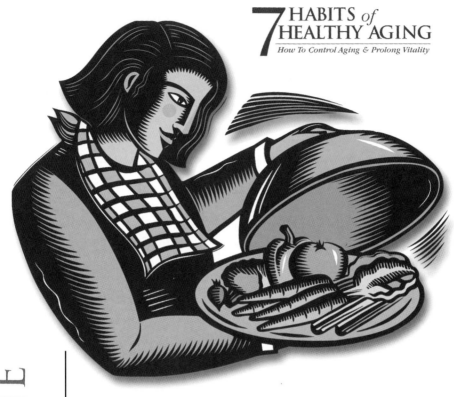

7 HABITS *of*
HEALTHY AGING
How To Control Aging & Prolong Vitality

CHAPTER ONE

HABIT #1 BALANCED EATING

Habit #1
Balanced Eating

KEY CONCEPT
A balanced meal is a meal that has all three of the major macronutrients present: carbohydrates, fats and protein. Each meal should consist of 15 grams of protein, 20 grams of wholesome complex carbohydrates and 6-7 grams of healthy oils, such as Omega 3 EFAs and/or monounsaturates.

Balanced eating habits have a direct influence on excess insulin production and the eventual condition known as sarcopenia (age-related loss of muscle).

Perhaps the most powerful tool in controlling the aging process and restoring vitality is to improve your lean body mass-to-body fat ratio by adding more muscle to your body. In order to accomplish this, two crucial hormones, insulin and glucagon, must be balanced through balancing protein, carbohydrate and fat ratios at each meal. A balanced meal is a meal that has all three of the major macronutrients present: carbohydrates, fats and protein. Each meal or snack should consist of 15 grams of quality protein, 20 grams of wholesome complex carbohydrates and 6-7 grams of healthy oils, like Omega 3 EFAs and/or monounsaturates. (See page 27 for additional information)

By balancing your meals and favorably influencing critical hormone pathways, you will experience noticeable improvement in the way you feel and the way your body looks. As an extra benefit, this process can literally reduce acute or chronic inflammatory conditions existing in your body.

When your intake of carbohydrates is excessive or too refined (sugar, alcohol, white flour, etc.) at any one meal, insulin is released to counter the resulting rapid rise in blood sugar. In most people, this results in a significant increase in the formation of fat, fatigue, mood swings and inflammation.

HOW THE BODY REACTS TO A BALANCED MEAL

Let's follow a balanced meal through the body to see how it affects insulin production. Insulin is directly impacted at all times by the type of food you put in your mouth.

1. Remember, a balanced meal is one that has all three of the major macronutrients present: carbohydrates, fats and protein. Each meal or snack should consist of 15 grams of quality protein, 20 grams of wholesome complex carbohydrates and 6-7 grams of healthy oils, like Omega 3 EFAs and/or monounsaturates. The process of digesting a balanced meal is also thermogenic. That means there is more energy required from the body to perform digestion on a balanced or complex meal, and, therefore, the body will also burn more calories.

2. Up to a four-hour period will ensue where small amounts of the digested food from the balanced meal will enter the portal vein (located between the small intestines and the liver) and enter the liver.

3. The glycemic index of the balanced meal (a rating of foods based on their blood glucose and insulin-raising potential) entering the portal vein triggers the pancreas to secrete insulin. The higher the sugar content of the meal, the higher the insulin secreted. If you eat a balanced meal, a low amount of insulin is released due to the complex nature of the meal.

4. The nutrients are sent to the liver for sorting. One of the liver's responsibilities is to tightly regulate how much sugar (glucose) passes through to the blood supply and on to the brain. A person's brain represents only three percent of his or her total body weight, yet it consumes as much as 20 percent of the available blood sugar. The brain is also a very strong trigger of muscle breakdown (sarcope nia). The muscle is then used for glucose, if sufficient amounts of blood glucose are not present in the bloodstream at all times.

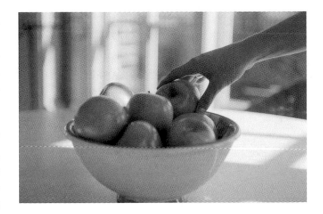

5. The relatively low amount of insulin secreted by the pancreas as a response to the balanced meal aids the liver in doing its job.

6. By eating balanced meals every time you put food in your mouth, you will keep the body working at its optimum and prevent sarcopenia and accelerated aging.

HOW THE BODY REACTS TO AN IMBALANCED MEAL
Imbalanced meals or snacks do not have a balanced ratio of carbohydrates, fats and proteins.

1. A meal or snack is eaten that is not balanced. It is either a pure refined carbohydrate, like a doughnut, or a "fat-free" snack. Due to the "refined" nature of the meal or snack, it is quickly broken down into sugar.

2. The sugar from the meal or snack leaves the small intestine and enters the portal vein with a very high glycemic index (a rating of foods based on their blood glucose and insulin-raising potential) that triggers the release of a high amount of insulin.

3. The insulin and sugar enter the liver with the high amount of insulin, alerting the liver to go into action.

4. Since the amount of sugar entering the liver is too high to pass through to the bloodstream and the brain, the liver converts the sugar into other forms of energy to "tightly regulate" the release of glucose to the bloodstream.

5. The liver can do the following with the "excess" sugar:
    a. use some of the sugar for immediate energy needs of the body.
    b. store some of the sugar in liver cells as glycogen for later energy needs.

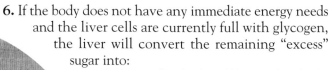

6. If the body does not have any immediate energy needs and the liver cells are currently full with glycogen, the liver will convert the remaining "excess" sugar into:

> ***a.*** cholesterol, which will be used to build hormones and cell membranes.
>
> > ***b.*** triglycerides, which are fatty acids that are used by most of the cells of the body for energy, or stored in fat cells that become the main "fat" of the body.

HOW YOUR BODY REACTS WHEN YOU SKIP MEALS

Insulin is indirectly increased by skipping meals or irregular eating habits.

1. Breakfast is skipped because you have no appetite or there is no time.

2. At some point midmorning, blood glucose levels drop to a point where the brain becomes concerned it may soon not have a sufficient supply to function properly.

3. The brain will not use stored fat (triglycerides) as an energy source except under extreme starvation conditions, so it has no choice but to create its own glucose supply.

4. Adrenaline and cortisol are stimulated to make new glucose for the brain by breaking down muscle through a process in the liver called gluconeogenesis. Keep in mind that the presence of adrenaline suppresses the appetite even further.

5. Since both adrenaline and cortisol are anti-insulin hormones, the next time you eat, the pancreas must secrete an extra amount of insulin to counteract the presence of these chemicals. This high level of insulin will be triggered even if the person eats only a small amount of carbohydrates. This constant overproduction of insulin, due to irregular eating habits, will contribute to hyperinsulenemia that eventually leads to insulin resistance, Syndrome X, and

Type II diabetes.

6. By eating breakfast and consuming four to six regular small meals throughout the day, you can lower your insulin levels, maintain normal blood sugar, slow down or stop muscle breakdown from sarcopenia, and prevent accelerated aging.

WHAT ARE CARBOHYDRATES?
Carbohydrates are chains of sugar molecules, classified as either simple or complex. Carbohydrates are found in both natural and man-made foods, such as whole grains, starchy vegetables, fruits, most dairy products, breads, cereals, pasta and sweets. Both complex carbohydrates (vegetables/grains) and simple carbohydrates (fruits/candy) are broken down in the digestive track to single-sugar molecules. Therefore, all carbohydrates are sugars.

HOW DOES THE BODY USE CARBOHYDRATES?
How your body utilizes the carbohydrates (sugars) you eat is based on the ratio of insulin to glucagon, the two main hormones made in the pancreas for nutritional distribution.

WHAT IS INSULIN?
Insulin is the fat-storage hormone. It is responsible for unloading nutrients (proteins, fats and sugar) in the bloodstream and putting them into the cells of the body. This process makes certain that the body is replenished and refueled, and blood-sugar levels are balanced, protecting the brain. Insulin also tells the liver that too much sugar has entered, and the liver reacts by increasing fat production from the incoming sugar, making cholesterol and triglycerides.

WHAT IS GLUCAGON?
Glucagon is an important hormone for mobilizing nutrients. Glucagon directs the liver to release sugar, which raises the levels of blood sugar available for the brain and body. Glucagon also directs the cells to release fat that can be used as energy and to release proteins that can be used as building materials.

The ratio between these two hormones, insulin and glucagon, determines whether food will be used as building materials or fuel, or stored as fat. If there is a higher proportion of glucagon, more food will be used as building materials or fuel. If there a higher proportion of insulin, more food will be stored as fat.

Glucagon is released in response to protein foods. Insulin is released in response to carbohydrates and some amino acids. Neither is released when nonstarchy vegetables like broccoli and fats are consumed. Therefore, if carbohydrates are eaten alone, the insulin-to-glucagon ratio is too high and excess food will be stored as fat.

If proteins are eaten alone, the insulin-to-glucagon ratio is too low, and lean body mass or muscle could be destroyed (sarcopenia). If fats or nonstarchy vegetables are eaten alone, there is no effect on the insulin-to-glucagon ratio.

If you follow the Balanced Eating Habit of proteins, fats and carbohydrates with every meal, you'll have a balanced insulin-to-glucagon ratio, which is the goal of Habit #1 and the Healthy Aging Program.

THE GLYCEMIC INDEX OF FOODS

In addition to eating carbohydrates or proteins alone, the insulin-to-glucagon ratio is also affected by the glycemic index of foods, a measure of how fast insulin rises in response to the amount of sugar entering the portal vein at any given moment. The faster sugar arrives, and the higher the amount of sugar entering the portal vein, the higher the glycemic index of that food. In general, simple sugars, such as candy and deserts, arrive faster than complex sugars, such as whole fruits and vegetables. Therefore, simple sugars have a higher glycemic index than complex carbohydrates.

Whole grains have a lower glycemic index than their refined counterparts. The fiber in the whole grain slows the rate of absorption of sugar into the system, lowering the insulin-to-glucagon ratio. The refining process, as in white rice or white bread, removes this protective coating of fiber.

WHY BALANCED EATING IS SO IMPORTANT

How you combine proteins, fats and carbohydrates is very important. If you eat only a baked potato for dinner, the glycemic index of that meal is higher than if you ate that potato with chicken and a salad. The reason is, carbohydrates enter the bloodstream much faster than proteins and fats. Carbohydrates cause insulin release, but they do not cause glucagon levels to go up.

When you eat excess carbohydrates or carbohydrates without protein and fat, the secretion of insulin is higher, and the secretion of glucagon is lower (high insulin-to-glucagon ratio). Consequently, the excess carbohydrates will mostly be stored as fat. When you eat protein and fat with carbohydrates, the secretion of insulin is lower and the secretion of glucagon is higher (low insulin-to-glucagon ratio). The result is that the food you ate will be used to rebuild the body or used as energy, not stored as fat.

Many people believe that eating protein and fat will cause you to get fat. Protein and fat actually lower the insulin-to-glucagon ratio, which will help prevent fat production and storage. Carbohydrates raise the insulin-to-glucagon ratio, which leads to fat production and storage.

INSULIN AND GLUCAGON HORMONES - THE BOTTOM LINE
The net effect of the insulin-to-glucagon ratio over time is that if you eat carbohydrates alone, the ratio will be too high and fat storage will occur. If you eat protein alone, the ratio will be too low and lean body mass will be destroyed. However, if you always practice Habit #1, Balanced Eating, making sure all meals contain protein, fats and carbohydrates, the ratio will be balanced and the body will maintain a Healthy Aging continuum.

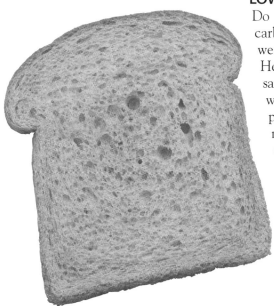

LOW CARBOHYDRATE DIETS
Do not go on a very low or "zero" gram carbohydrate diet in order to see faster weight loss. The primary goal of the Healthy Aging Program is to prevent sarcopenia (age related loss of muscle). A weight loss of more than one to two pounds per week is an indication of muscle loss. In order to prevent sarcopenia, you must keep insulin levels balanced. When insulin levels are kept too low or are out of balance, through over exercising or low carbohydrates, you will trigger sarcopenia and may begin to suffer from depression, fatigue, insomnia and bone loss. This will undermine your goal of controlling the aging process and prolonging vitality.

HEALTHY AGING INCLUDES A HEALTHY APPETITE
As you follow the Healthy Aging Program, you may find that you feel more hungry. This is often a problem for those who have been forcing themselves to follow a low-calorie diet. Chronic dieting often times turns off hunger signs. Feeling hungry again is a good sign of improved health. Hunger indicates your metabolism is improving and your brain needs vital energy. You should eat when you are hungry, but make sure that you follow Habit #1, Balanced Eating, by always eating proteins, fats and complex carbohydrates at every meal.

CUT BACK ON REFINED SUGAR - "EMPTY CARBOHYDRATES"
Be sure to cut back on low-nutrient carbohydrates by eliminating white bread and pasta, candy, juices, crackers, bagels and such from your diet. It's a known scientific fact that your body has trouble burning fat when your insulin levels are elevated, and eating these types of "empty" carbohydrates causes a spike in insulin levels.

CONSUME HIGH QUALITY MEAL-REPLACEMENT SHAKES
With today's busy lifestyles, it's hard to find the time to prepare multiple, nutritionally balanced, complete whole-food meals. Fortunately, certain meal-replacement shakes offer a simple solution to this complex problem.

Whole foods should be the cornerstone of your nutritional regime. Eating a diet primarily of clean whole-food carbohydrates, protein and fat sources requires your body to use more energy for digestion, absorption, and disposal of the ingested food, which ultimately contributes to fat loss.

Good quality meal-replacement shakes play a very important role in healthy aging because they provide exact portions of high-quality protein, energy-rich carbohydrates and fats, plus important vitamins and minerals, without excess sugar. Try to make whole foods comprise at least two or three of your five daily meals (as explained in Chapter 2) and then fill the remaining two or three with a high quality meal replacement

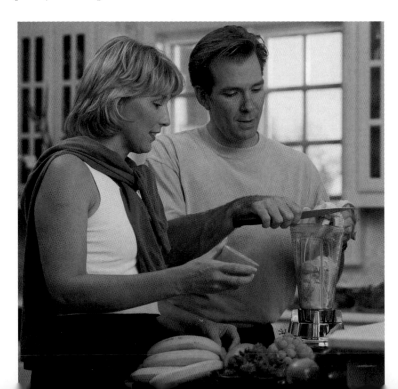

EAT MORE FIBER
Fiber helps speed up fat loss by preventing the entry of some carbohydrates into the bloodstream, which in turn slows the entry of sugar into the blood. High levels of sugar or glucose in the bloodstream spike insulin levels, which slow fat burning and may lead to muscle loss. Good sources of fiber include bran, beans and brown rice, as well as green vegetables such as broccoli, asparagus and spinach. Try to consume fibrous vegetables with at least two of your five daily meals.

CONSUME MORE PROTEIN
Most experts today agree that protein consumption is one of the most important aspects of an overall health program. Studies show that maintaining a diet of proper protein increases the muscle-growing benefits of resistance training. As you age or lose fat, you need even more protein because your body burns more protein with a reduced basal metabolic rate. Protein drinks and meal-replacement shakes can help in this area, since consuming enough protein each day can be difficult with whole foods alone.

Ensuring adequate intake of quality proteins with each meal stimulates the release of glucagon, a very favorable hormone with respect to improving the muscle-to-fat ratio, and is also helpful in increasing energy and endurance. Like carbohydrates, however, too many proteins in your diet can favor inflammation and other undesirable consequences. Your daily protein requirement needs to be calculated specifically by considering your current level of lean body mass and your exercise activity level. (Refer to your Personal Program Recommendations and Habit #2.)

INCREASE HEALTHY FATS AND OILS
Certain fats are very important in regulating your metabolism. Eliminating them from your diet will tend to increase unwanted weight. Healthy fats, especially Omega-3 EFAs, possess thermogenic properties and will help your body produce heat by burning fat. Make sure you eat foods rich in the healthy essential fatty acids (EFAs) such as cold-water fish, like salmon, sardines, mackerel and trout. In addition, consume a good supply of EFA-rich oil like flax seed or hemp oil by adding the oil to salads or meal-replacement shakes.

POLYUNSATURATED (Heat damages these fats-Do not use for cooking)
Corn oil, Essential Fatty Acids (borage, flaxseed, primrose), herring oil, menhaden (fish) oil, salmon oil, sardine oil, sesame seed oil and wheat germ oil.

MONOUNSATURATED (Suitable for cooking)
Almond oil, apricot kernel oil, avocado oil, canola oil, grape seed oil, hazelnut oil, mustard oil, oat oil, olive oil, peanut oil and rice oil

FREQUENTLY ASKED QUESTIONS ABOUT INSULIN

WHY IS INSULIN BALANCE SO IMPORTANT?

Insulin is the major fuel-regulation hormone for the body. It is secreted in the bloodstream when blood glucose (sugar) goes up. Blood glucose is the end product of digesting carbohydrates. Insulin promotes the storage of carbohydrates in the form of glycogen in the liver and muscles, or as fat in the fat cells. Insulin prevents the breakdown of stored body fat and, thereby, keeps a person fat. In fact, the reason obesity is so high in our society is that most Americans spend each and every day with insulin levels that are far too high, because of overindulging in too many carbohydrates and not enough protein and healthy fats. High insulin levels, called hyperinsulinemia, are caused by a hormonal imbalance. When hormones are out of balance, a person may be plagued with recurrent hunger and cravings, mood swings, lethargy, obesity around the midsection, loss of endurance and power, shortened life span, insulin resistance, Syndrome X, diabetes, heart disease, cancer, a suppressed immune system, and many other chronic diseases.

HOW DO I KEEP INSULIN LEVELS BALANCED?

Nearly 80 to 90 percent of the control over blood sugar and insulin production centers around balanced eating habits; the remaining 10 percent is a regular exercise program. What you put in your mouth is absolutely the most important factor in keeping insulin levels in the ideal range for fat burning, muscle building and optimal health. By following the 7 Habits of Healthy Aging Program and consuming five to six small meals per day with the right balance of healthy fats, protein and low-glycemic carbohydrates, you'll be on the right path to balance.

WHAT TYPE OF BALANCED EATING LOWERS INSULIN LEVELS?

The key to low insulin levels is to eat five to six small meals a day, consisting of a balance of protein, carbohydrate, and fat. Lean meats and low-fat fish such as tuna, swordfish and sea bass are good sources of protein and the healthy fats your body needs. Most of the carbohydrates you eat should come from fruits, vegetables and whole grains, which are low on the glycemic index and won't dramatically affect blood sugar. Stay away from processed grains and "fat-free" foods since they are usually full of sugar, which really increases blood sugar and insulin levels. Eat all carbohydrates with some fat and protein. This will make you feel fuller, while slowing the movement of glucose into the bloodstream.

HOW DOES EATING HEALTHY OILS
LOWER INSULIN LEVELS AND BURN BODY FAT?

Monounsaturated fats, like olive oil, almonds, avocados and canola oil, play a critical role in controlling insulin secretion by slowing the rate that carbohydrates are digested and enter your bloodstream. This slowdown enables your body to more effectively tap into your stored body fat for energy. Contrary to what has been told over the past 10 years, healthy fat in your diet is very important to your health and aids in fat loss. Healthy fats should be incorporated into each of your five to six meals daily. Healthy diets must have adequate amounts of essential fatty acids, since these are fats your body cannot make. These essen-

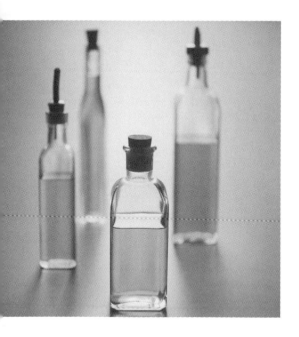

tial fatty acids include both the Omega-3s and Omega-6s. They are very important, since they are the building blocks of important hormones that regulate your essential biological functions. Usually, you'll get plenty of Omega-6 fatty acids from low-fat protein sources, such as chicken and tuna. But unless you eat a lot of cold-water fish like salmon, you probably have a hard time getting enough Omega-3s. If this is the case, you should take fish-oil supplements because those Omega-3 fatty acids help control your insulin levels. And don't forget vitamin E, which helps the Omega-3s work even better. Don't use saturated fat, and use sparingly the Omega-6 polyunsaturated fats found in most vegetable oils and vegetable shortening.

HOW LONG DO I HAVE TO KEEP MY INSULIN BALANCED?

Insulin balance is not a short-term goal but a nutrition plan for your entire life. It is a way of living that will bring you a longer life packed with vitality, wellness and optimal health. It won't happen overnight, but once you have established the 7 Habits lifestyle for a while, the positive benefits will make it worth the effort to eat wholesome, balanced meals most of the time.

HOW DOES EXERCISE LOWER INSULIN LEVELS?

When you are insulin resistant, your pancreas has to produce more insulin to maintain normal blood sugar levels, and more insulin means more body fat. Both cardio and strength-building exercises have been shown to reverse insulin resistance. The more fat you burn through exercise, the more sensitive you become to the insulin your body produces. As body fat disappears and muscle mass develops, your insulin resistance diminishes, which will take a huge burden off your pancreas, requiring less insulin throughout the day. The greater your sensitivity to insulin, the more effective you become at removing sugar from your blood and keeping your blood sugar and insulin levels in a healthy range.

HOW DOES KEEPING INSULIN LEVELS LOW KEEP ME LEAN?

Body fat accumulates from a combination of too many refined carbohydrates, like white bread, cookies, and sweets, and not enough balanced eating and exercise. When you eat complex carbohydrates that don't trigger high levels of insulin and add a regular exercise program, your insulin and blood sugar levels remain balanced. Some of the immediate benefits are a decrease in appetite and cravings for the refined sugars. In addition, your body turns to its storage of fat rather than glycogen for energy, and you begin to lose body fat while sparing muscle mass.

HOW DO LOW INSULIN LEVELS ADD MUSCLE?

Research shows that diets higher in carbohydrates and lower in protein tend to increase insulin secretion and produce a negative nitrogen balance. On the other hand, a diet that is balanced with more protein tends to keep insulin levels low and maintains a positive nitrogen balance. A negative nitrogen balance means that you are breaking down your muscle to provide energy for your body. A positive nitrogen balance, on the other hand, means that you are building muscle mass. If you practice a balanced eating program, as suggested in the 7 Habits of Healthy Aging, and strive to keep your insulin balanced, you may not only spare muscle loss but may also gain increased mass.

WHAT IS THE RELATIONSHIP BETWEEN INSULIN LEVELS AND HEART DISEASE?

Hyperinsulinemia, or an elevated fasting insulin level, is one of the most powerful predictors of heart disease. It occurs as a result of the development of insulin resistance from dietary habits that encourage indiscriminate, uncontrolled eating of a high-carbohydrate diet. Constant increases in blood sugar due to imbalanced eating makes insulin less able to do its job and requires more of it to meet daily needs. High insulin levels slowly cripple the immune system, increase body fat and blood pressure, and trigger more serious degenerative diseases including the number one cause of death in the United States: heart disease. The type of carbohydrates eaten affects blood sugar levels and, therefore, how much insulin the body produces. By eating a balanced diet and exercising, you can improve your chances of preventing heart disease.

HOW LONG DOES IT TAKE TO BALANCE INSULIN LEVELS?

Of course, every individual is different. But in many cases, in as short as four to seven days of following the 7 Habits of Healthy Aging Program, you can begin to balance your blood sugar and insulin levels. Within two to three weeks, you may no longer have feelings of hunger, cravings and mood swings. In addition, you should notice a marked improvement in strength, begin to see a reduction in body fat, and experience an overall feeling of well-being.

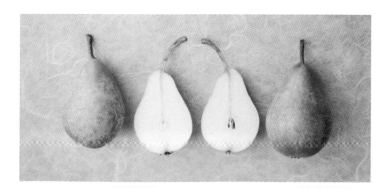

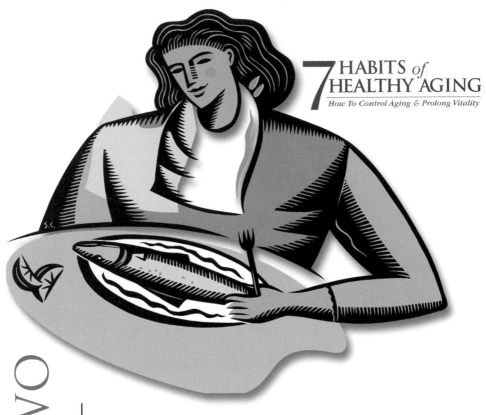

7 HABITS *of* HEALTHY AGING

How To Control Aging & Prolong Vitality

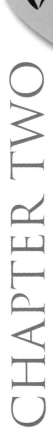

CHAPTER TWO

Habit #2
Eating Frequency

KEY CONCEPT

Insulin is increased by skipping meals or following irregular eating habits, which can lead to an increase in body fat and decrease in muscle. Determine your daily protein requirement and spread your meals evenly throughout the day, consuming approximately 15 grams of protein with each meal, whether it is real food, a meal-replacement shake or a nutrition bar. If the number of meals required per day proves to be too many for your lifestyle, then you may double up at one or more meals by consuming up to 30 grams of protein, 40 grams of complex carbohydrates and 12-14 grams of healthy oils per meal. Never eat less than five meals that contain 15 grams of protein each, in order to maintain a minimum of 800 calories per day.

Improving your eating frequency will allow body fat to be mobilized as energy rather than be stored as fat.

Poor or infrequent eating habits have an influence on excess insulin production and the eventual condition known as sarcopenia (aged-related muscle loss) through the stimulation of the hormones adrenaline and cortisol.

A lifestyle of irregular eating habits contributes to increased insulin production, increased body fat and decreased muscle.

Skipping breakfast, for instance, or only eating two meals a day does not provide enough nutrition to prevent muscle loss and fat deposition. Three or four meals are significantly better than two. Five meals per day would be better still. It's permissible to regard two or three of your meals as "snacks," provided they comprise sufficient ratios of proteins, carbohydrates and healthy oils.

It's important to spread your meals evenly throughout the day. Your blood sugar and insulin levels and, thus, your energy level will be controlled; you'll get available protein in small amounts to support muscle growth and recovery. Most importantly, this type of improved eating frequency will allow body fat to be mobilized as an energy source rather than be stored on the waist or hips.

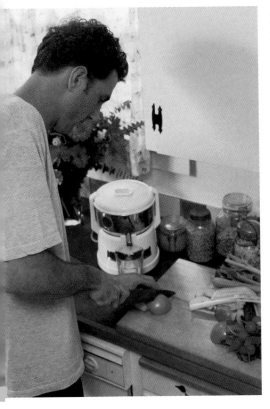

ARE YOU A GRAZER OR BINGER?

Nature offers extreme examples of "grazers" and "bingers." For example, deer graze; they eat small amounts consistently throughout their waking hours, and most deer are low-fat, high-muscle animals. Bears, on the other hand, eat like most humans do; they go extended periods of time without eating and then "binge" or eat large amounts of food. Consequently, bears like some humans, have a large amount of body fat. The lesson to learn is, if you want to be leaner and more muscular, you need to graze, not binge.

Stick to the tried-and-true, whole-food sources of protein such as skinless chicken breasts, fish, lean red meat, egg whites and whole eggs. Select your carbohydrates carefully, with an emphasis on vegetables, yams, baked potatoes and starches such as rice and pasta, without fattening sauces.

Simply by providing your body with a consistent, frequent and appropriate supply of protein, carbohydrates and healthy oils, you'll eliminate your body's need to store fat.

If you eat infrequently or skip meals, your body perceives a "famine" situation, and your endocrine system, through the release of hormones like insulin, slows, stops or even reverses muscle growth

DETERMINE YOUR DAILY PROTEIN REQUIREMENT

In order to determine your daily protein requirement and establish a proper eating habit frequency, ask your healthcare provider to conduct a body composition analysis to determine your current level of muscle mass.

With information about your body composition and your current level of exercise activity, your healthcare provider can help you calculate your daily protein requirement. Divide the amount of daily protein required in grams by 15. For example, if your protein

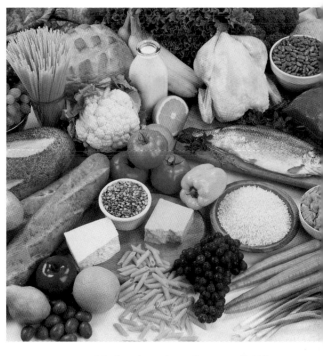

requirement per day were 75 grams, you would divide it by 15 to get 5. This number represents the number of small meals you should eat per day. At each of these five meals, you should consume the equivalent of 15 grams of quality protein, 20 grams of wholesome complex carbohydrates, and no more than 6-7 grams of quality monounsaturated fats or Omega-3 rich oils. Never eat less than five of these small meals per day to ensure that you maintain at least 800 calories per day.

Remember, an easy way to fulfill several of the required meals each day is to use a high quality, ratio-balanced powdered meal replacement that only requires the addition of water. Be sure to look for a product that contains approximately 15 grams of protein, 20 grams of low glycemic carbohydrates and 1 gram of fat.

If your daily requirement of protein is 75 grams, you may choose three servings of a meal-replacement powder, 3 oz. of salmon and 2 oz. of chicken breast (15g each) to meet your protein requirement for that day.

For each 15-gram portion of protein, choose a 20-gram portion of complex carbohydrates and 6-7 grams of essential fatty acids or monounsaturated oils.

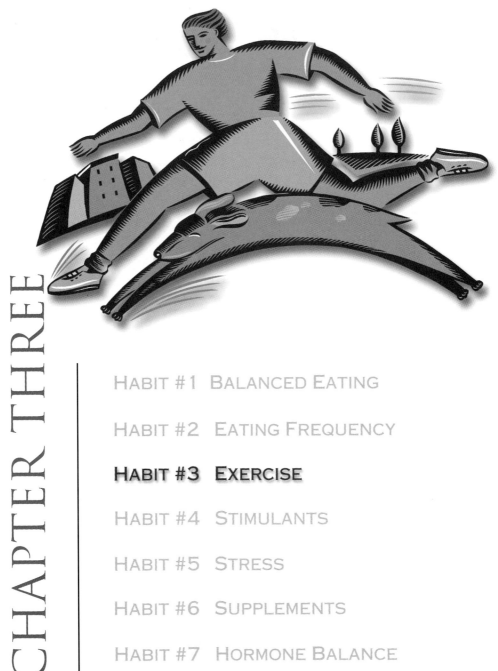

7 HABITS *of* HEALTHY AGING
How To Control Aging & Prolong Vitality

CHAPTER THREE

Habit #3
Exercise

KEY CONCEPT
Muscle is youth! Regular exercise, along with proper diet, will increase your chances of staying well longer and slowing down the aging process. Other benefits of regular exercise are increased energy, stamina and a better body shape. Follow one of the three exercise plans: Plan #1 Low Fit, Plan #2 Moderately Fit or Plan #3 Maintaining Fitness.

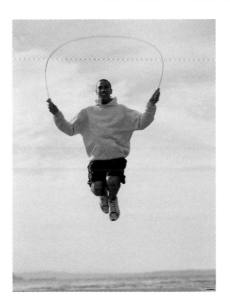

Exercise has a direct influence on insulin and sarcopenia (age-related loss of muscle) and is a vital component of the 7 Habits of Healthy Aging Program. The exercise programs recommended in this chapter will help decrease insulin, reverse insulin resistance and, therefore, help control the aging process and prolong vitality.

DIET AND EXERCISE ARE INTERRELATED

Top researchers on aging define a youthful person both as someone who has a large oxygen transport system and a large amount of lean muscle. Both are highly accurate measures of your biological age based on widely accepted scientific tests. Researchers in the field of aging call these tests "biomarkers" of aging. They believe that these tests are much more reliable indicators of the "age you function at" than your "age in years."

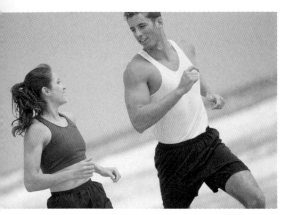

These same researchers indicate that diet and exercise are interrelated when it comes to slowing down or reversing the aging process. Regular exercise, plus a proper diet geared toward specific age-related needs, are a powerful duo. This combination increases your chances of staying well longer and retarding the progression of accelerated aging.

A proper diet and little to no exercise won't help slow the aging process anymore than avid exercise and a bad diet. If you want to maintain vitality, the answer is allegiance to both: good dietary principles plus regular resistance, cardio and flexibility exercises.

Muscle is youth! Every decade from the age of 40, the average person loses about 6.6 pounds of muscle. It may not be apparent, since the size of the arm or leg often remains the same size as when you were younger, but fat has replaced muscle. The less muscle a person has, the less they can eat without getting fat, because they have less active tissue to burn calories, whether at rest or during exercise. The average 25-year-old man is 18 percent body fat, but by age 65 he has 38 percent body fat! Much of that fat gain is due to the loss of vital, active, calorie-burning muscle.

With exercise, you can increase your daily carbohydrate intake. However, you cannot reduce your carbohydrate consumption to a dangerously low level to justify not exercising. Severe restriction of carbohydrate consumption will lead to hormone imbalances. If you do lose "weight," it will be muscle, not fat, which leads to further metabolic aging. You cannot reverse accelerated metabolic aging by only changing your eating habits.

Even though most people know the health benefits of exercise, many remark how difficult it is to get motivated. Exercise often becomes the lowest priority. On the other hand, those who begin and stay with an exercise program are generally the most enthusiastic advocates and are likely to make exercise a high priority. The reason is, those who begin an exercise program soon discover that exercise is one sure way to improve the overall quality of their life.

Habit #3 in this book is dedicated to ACTION. The following pages focus on exercises that will markedly improve the chances that your body will age at a much slower rate than chronology would normally dictate. By adhering faithfully to one of the three Healthy Aging Plans outlined, you may expect to experience renewed vigor, improved musculature and more stamina, not to mention newfound flexibility and strength. Many people also report an emotional, as well as a physical, improvement from following the entire 7 Habits of Healthy Aging Program.

HEALTHY AGING EXERCISE DISCLAIMER-PLEASE READ FIRST!

It is imperative to consult your primary healthcare provider before starting any anti-aging healthcare or new workout program. According to the President's Council on Physical Fitness, you should consult with a doctor if you have any medical concerns, particularly heart disease, high blood pressure, elevated cholesterol levels, frequent dizzy spells, extreme breathlessness after mild exertion, arthritis or other bone problems, severe muscular or ligament problems, back problems, obesity, or a family history of such diseases. If you started this program as part of your healthcare provider's recommendation and have not disclosed any of the noted concerns, do so prior to starting this or any other healthcare or fitness program. If you have multiple health problems, consider starting with an exercise rehabilitation center. Your healthcare provider can advise you which facility in your area is best for you.

Regardless of which Healthy Aging Plan you begin with, always maintain a regular log. A personal program log and complete instructions for its use have been provided at the end of this book, (Appendix D, pages 120-124) to help you record and monitor your progress and achieve success!

CALCULATING YOUR HEALTHY AGING HEART RATE ZONE

In addition to estimating your overall **Actual**Age™, you will also need to estimate the target heart rate zone you should maintain while performing any of the exercises recommended.

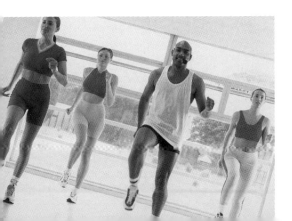

Typically, your target heart rate zone is between 50 percent and 85 percent of your maximum heart rate, which is the maximum number of times your heart can beat in a minute. The three possible target heart rate zones and how to estimate which one is right for you are as follows:

50% *of Your Maximum:* If your **Actual**Age™ score is 10 years
or more above your chronological age.

60% *of Your Maximum:* If your **Actual**Age™ score is one
to nine years above your chronological age.

70% *of Your Maximum:* If your **Actual**Age™ score is your
chronological age or below.

To calculate your target heart rate zone, use the steps listed below:

A) Estimate your maximum heart rate: 220 minus your age =_____.

B) Determine your lower limit exercise heart rate by multiplying your
maximum heart rate by 0.5.

C) Determine your medium limit exercise heart rate by multiplying your
maximum heart rate by 0.6.

D) Determine your maximum limit exercise heart rate by multiplying your
maximum heart rate by 0.7.

E) Your exercise heart rate range is between your upper and lower limits.

HEALTHY AGING WALKING TEST TO GET YOU STARTED
One of the best ways to stay motivated is to measure your progress. With this in
mind, we want to start you off with a very simple walking test.

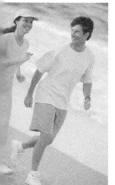

QUARTER-MILE WALKING TEST
• Mark off a quarter-mile course using landmarks, like telephone
poles, fire hydrants or a specific store as your guide. The distance
does not have to be exact as long as you always perform this test
in the same place, so you're always consistent.

• Walk the course as rapidly as you can, timing yourself using a
watch with a second hand or a stopwatch. At the end of the
course, stop and immediately measure your pulse rate for 30
seconds, or have your exercise partner measure it for you.

• Ideally you should repeat this self-test once every two weeks,
during weeks 3, 5, 7, 9, 11, 13 and 15.

• Each time, walk the course as fast as you can and monitor your pulse for half a minute. As you become better trained, this test will become easier and easier, and your pulse rate will be lower and lower. Conditioned people have efficient cardiovascular systems. It takes progressively more exertion to make their hearts pump harder.

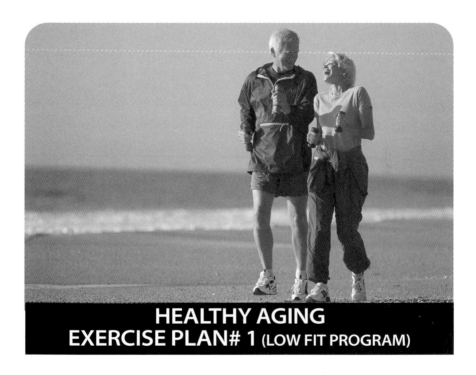

HEALTHY AGING
EXERCISE PLAN# 1 (LOW FIT PROGRAM)

(Actual Age™ **measures 10 years or more above chronological age)**
Your **Actual**Age™ results indicated an overall **Actual**Age™ for you of 10 or more years older than your chronological age. Before you become depressed about where you're starting, know this: research shows that the single best predictor of how much gain an individual will make during an exercise program is his or her baseline fitness. This puts those who start in Exercise Plan #1 in the enviable position of having more to look forward to than those folks who are already in pretty good shape.

In Exercise Plan #1, you will focus your attention for the next four weeks exclusively on a cardiovascular aerobic exercise program, with no muscular conditioning scheduled. Following is the Exercise Plan #1 four-week aerobic program. When you finish with Exercise Plan #1, you should immediately schedule an appointment with your healthcare provider to receive another evaluation and clearance to begin Exercise Plan #2.

EXERCISE PLAN #1 FOUR-WEEK AEROBIC PROGRAM

WEEK 1

Day 1   Divide your exercise walk into two separate sessions of 10 minutes each, keeping your total time to no more than 20 minutes.

Day 2   Follow yesterday's session, again for 20 minutes, and be sure not to exceed your calculated target heart rate zone.

Day 3   Walk or perform some other form of aerobic exercise in two separate sessions for a total of 20 minutes.

Day 4   Repeat yesterday's aerobic program again for only 20 minutes.

Day 5   Rest today, if you feel you need it. If not, walk or perform some other aerobic exercise for 10 minutes only.

Day 6   Today conduct two 15-minute aerobic sessions of your choice or three 10-minute sessions.

Day 7   Repeat yesterday's aerobic program conducting either two 15-minute sessions or three 10-minute sessions.

WEEK 2

Day 8   Today, perform two 15-minute walking or other aerobic sessions.

Day 9   Repeat yesterday's aerobic program, conducting two 15-minute sessions.

Day 10 Rest Day

Day 11 Today, for 20-consecutive minutes, either walk or perform some other aerobic exercise. Be sure not to exceed your calculated target heart rate zone.

Day 12 Repeat yesterday's aerobic program again for 20 minutes.

Day 13 Once again, conduct your aerobic exercise of choice for 20 minutes.

Day 14 Today, walk or conduct any aerobic exercise for at least 20 minutes. You should be able to push yourself harder and still stay within your target heart rate.

WEEK 3

Day 15 Walk or conduct any other aerobic exercise for 20 minutes without stopping. Increase your intensity.

Day 16 Repeat yesterday's aerobic program, again for 20 minutes.

Day 17 Rest Day

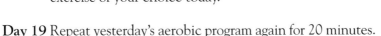

Day 18 Perform 20-minutes of continuous aerobic exercise of your choice today.

Day 19 Repeat yesterday's aerobic program again for 20 minutes.

Day 20 20 minutes of continuous aerobic exercise of your choice today.

Day 21 Repeat yesterday's aerobic program again for 20 minutes.

WEEK 4

Day 22 This week you will learn how to conduct the 25-Minute Interval Aerobics Workout. You will conduct your aerobic activity of choice for 20 minutes without stopping, plus a five-minute cool down period.

You'll start with a two-minute initial phase where you perform the aerobic activity of your choice at a level 5 intensity for you, on a scale of 1-10, with 1 being little effort and 10 being maximum effort.

After two minutes at a level 5, increase your effort to a level 6 for one minute, then increase your effort to a level 7 for one minute, then increase your effort to a level 8 for one minute, then once again increase your effort to a level 9 for one final minute.

After a full minute at level 9, drop your intensity down to level 6. Repeat this pattern three times, which will consume 18 minutes. After the 18th minute, increase the intensity from 9 to a maximum intensity of 10 for one minute, then for the last or the 20th minute, return to level 5, your original starting point.

Stay at level 5 for two minutes of cool down, than drop to level 3 for three additional minutes of cool down, or a total of five minutes. (Refer to the "25-minute Interval Aerobics Workout Schedule" on the next page).

25- MINUTE INTERVAL AEROBICS WORKOUT SCHEDULE

Minutes 1 & 2	Level 5
Minutes 3	Level 6
Minutes 4	Level 7
Minutes 5	Level 8
Minutes 6	Level 9
Minutes 7	Level 6
Minutes 8	Level 7
Minutes 9	Level 8
Minutes 10	Level 9
Minutes 11	Level 6
Minutes 12	Level 7
Minutes 13	Level 8
Minutes 14	Level 9
Minutes 15	Level 6
Minutes 16	Level 7
Minutes 17	Level 8
Minutes 18	Level 9
Minutes 19	Level 10
Minutes 20	Level 5
Minutes 21	Level 5
Minutes 22	Level 3
Minutes 23	Level 3
Minutes 24 & 25	Level 3

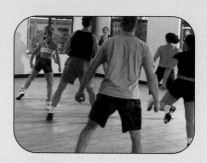

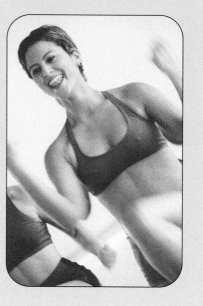

Day 23 Repeat yesterday's aerobic program again for 25 minutes.

Day 24 25 minutes of continuous aerobic exercise of your choice today.

Day 25 Repeat yesterday's aerobic program again for 25 minutes.

Day 26 Rest Day

Day 27 Perform 25 minutes of continuous aerobic exercise of your choice today.

Day 28 Repeat yesterday's aerobic program again for 25 minutes.

The last four-weeks of Exercise Plan #1 aerobic exercise offer proof that a person who measures 10 years or more older than their chronological age can respond to exercise in remarkable ways. Remember, at any age, you can increase your functional capacity. Healthy Aging Exercise Plan #1 has given you added strength and cardio endurance.

Research shows that conditioned people who want to maintain their fitness level must keep exercising. When conditioned people stop training, they lose what they've gained at a much faster rate than they gained it. This stands to reason. The more you have, the more you stand to lose.

Now that you've finished with Healthy Aging Exercise Plan #1, you should immediately receive an **Actual**Age™ re-test and, with your new results, begin Exercise Plan #2.

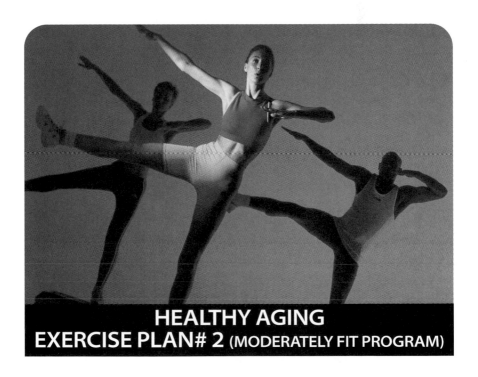

**HEALTHY AGING
EXERCISE PLAN# 2 (MODERATELY FIT PROGRAM)**

(**Actual**Age™ **measures one to nine years above chronological age**)
Your **Actual**Age™ results indicated an overall **Actual**Age™ for you of one to nine years older than your chronological age, or you have just finished the Healthy Aging Exercise Plan #1 and are now ready to continue with Exercise Plan #2.

This 12-week program is designed to both lose fat and build muscle. This program includes cardiovascular training, flexibility exercises, and strength training or resistance exercises.

EXERCISE PLAN #2 - CARDIOVASCULAR TRAINING

The 25-minute Interval Aerobics Workout outlined in Exercise Plan #1 should be conducted three days a week. If you did not participate in Exercise Plan #1, review the fourth week of Exercise Plan #1, which details how to conduct short duration, high-intensity interval aerobics.

Many people believe that low-intensity, long duration aerobic training will burn more body fat. New research shows that high-intensity exercise, like the type suggested in the Interval Aerobics Workout, may burn up to 50 percent more fat and speed up your metabolism. This type of aerobics program is not as dependent upon how many calories you burn during the exercise as how many will be burned for you up to an hour after the exercise.

To maximize fat loss with the Interval Aerobics Workout, it is recommended that you perform the exercises first thing in the morning on an empty stomach and not eat for one hour after the exercise.

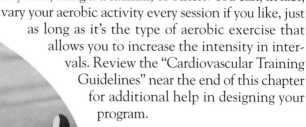

You may choose any aerobic activity like walking, jogging, riding a stationary bike, using a treadmill, or others. You can, in fact, vary your aerobic activity every session if you like, just as long as it's the type of aerobic exercise that allows you to increase the intensity in intervals. Review the "Cardiovascular Training Guidelines" near the end of this chapter for additional help in designing your program.

EXERCISE PLAN #2 - FLEXIBILITY/ STRETCHING EXERCISES

Stretching will reduce your body's workload in most daily activities by removing tightness, so you can swing your limbs more freely.

Stretching transports oxygen to sore muscles and quickly removes toxins from muscles, so recovery from exercise or sports activities is faster. We tend to do activities day in and day out that are very muscle specific, so we lose our elasticity in those muscles we don't use.

For example, many people's hips are almost entirely locked up. In a lot of cases, people mistake this condition for aging and simply slow down and limit their movements. Stretching, especially in the lower body, can unlock the hips, creating more of a free-floating pelvis by unbinding the connective tissue that so tightly constricts movement with age.

After your aerobics training, three days a week, you should conduct the Healthy Aging Stretching Workout. Review the "Stretching Routine" near the end of this chapter, paying particular attention to the five key points to maximize the workout. The entire upper and lower body program can be conducted in five to 10 minutes, after you become familiar with the 10 different recommended stretches.

The Healthy Aging Stretching Workout can also be used as a monitoring system for your flexibility, balance and strength. Stretching one group of muscles at a time allows you to specifically feel whether or not they're tight. If a group of muscles are continuously tight, this might indicate the muscles are either being overworked or compensating for another muscle group that's either weak or inflexible.

Your healthcare provider can use this stretching workout feedback as a monitoring system to counsel you on how to bring your flexibility and strength into balance. With this information, he or she will recommend any changes you need to make in the stretches you conduct or the stretching schedule. Review the "Flexibility Exercise/Stretching Guidelines" near the end of this chapter for additional help in designing your program.

EXERCISE PLAN #2 - STRENGTH TRAINING

Three days a week, perform strength training using weight machines, free weights or resistance training. Always warm up prior to any strength training routine. Refer to page 58 to learn "How to Estimate 80 Percent of Your One Repetition Maximum (1RM)," and see the more detailed explanation at the end of this chapter.

Alternate your schedule each week as follows:

Week 1: Upper Body, Lower Body, Upper Body
Week 2: Lower Body, Upper Body, Lower Body

Upper Body: Back, Chest, Shoulders, Biceps and Triceps
Choose two exercises for each of the upper body parts listed and complete the
following: three sets of 6-8 repetitions at 80% of 1RM for each body part.

Lower Body: Quadriceps, Hamstrings, Calves and Abdominals.
Choose two exercises for each of the lower body parts listed and complete the
following: three sets of 6-8 repetitions at 80% of 1RM for each body part.

HOW TO ESTIMATE 80 PERCENT OF YOUR
ONE REPETITION MAXIMUM (80% 1RM)
When doing a bench press, if you can lift the weight more than twelve times, it's
too light or below 80 percent of your 1RM. If, on the other hand, you can only
lift the weight eight times or less, it's too heavy or higher than 80 percent of your
1RM. The ideal estimate of 80% 1RM would have you lifting the weight
between nine to 10 repetitions, with repetition eight being difficult, repetition
nine being very difficult, and repetition 10 creating failure.

TYPICAL UPPER BODY WORKOUT

• **Back**	Lat-Pull Downs	3 sets of 6-8 repetitions at 80% 1RM
• **Chest**	Chest Press	3 sets of 6-8 repetitions at 80% 1RM
• **Shoulders**	Shoulder Press	3 sets of 6-8 repetitions at 80% 1RM
• **Biceps**	Curls	3 sets of 6-8 repetitions at 80% 1RM
• **Triceps**	Triceps Press	3 sets of 6-8 repetitions at 80% 1RM

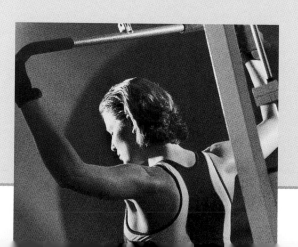

TYPICAL LOWER BODY

- **Quadriceps** Leg Press 3 sets of 6-8 repetitions at 80% 1RM
- **Hamstrings** Leg Curl 3 sets of 6-8 repetitions at 80% 1RM
- **Calves** Calf Raises 3 sets of 6-8 repetitions at 80% 1RM
- **Abdominal** Crunches 3 sets of 6-8 repetitions at 80% 1RM

Review the "Strength Training Guidelines" near the end of this chapter for help in designing your own program.

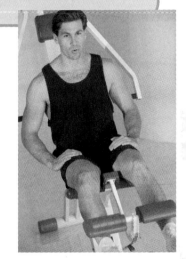

SUMMARY: HEALTHY AGING EXERCISE PLAN #2

Following is a typical Exercise Plan #2 weekly schedule. In this example, the upper body is getting exercised two times. Be sure, on the following week, to switch and exercise the lower body two times. Flexibility/stretching exercises should be done on the cardiovascular days, after your aerobic workout. Keep the intensity of the strength-training program at three sets of 6-8 repetitions at 80 percent of 1RM.

EXERCISE PLAN #2 WEEKLY GUIDE

Monday	Upper Body Strength Training
Tuesday	25 Minutes of Aerobics plus Flexibility/Stretching Exercises
Wednesday	Lower Body Strength Training
Thursday	25 Minutes of Interval Aerobics plus Flexibility/Stretching Exercises
Friday	Upper Body Strength Training
Saturday	25 minutes of Aerobics plus Flexibility/Stretching Exercises
Sunday	Rest

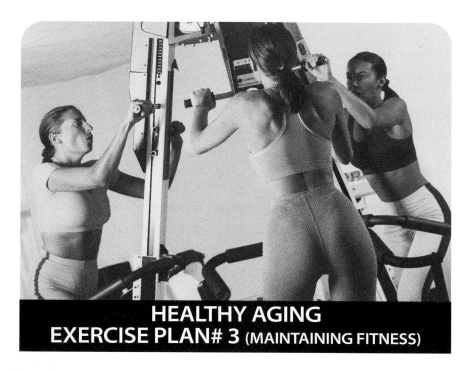

HEALTHY AGING
EXERCISE PLAN# 3 (MAINTAINING FITNESS)

(**Actual**Age™ equals chronological age or lower)
Your **Actual**Age™ results indicated an overall **Actual**Age™ for you at your chronological age or below. You either measured this way initially, or successfully reduced your **Actual**Age™ score by following the Exercise Plan #1 or #2. Either way, Exercise Plan #3 is an aerobic, strength and flexibility maintenance program to use for life, to prevent you from backsliding to a low or moderately fit condition.

EXERCISE PLAN #3 - CARDIOVASCULAR TRAINING

Conduct the 25-minute Interval Aerobics Workout outlined in Exercise Plan #1, three days a week. (If you did not participate in Exercise Plan #1, review the fourth week of Exercise Plan #1, which details how to conduct short duration, high intensity interval aerobics.) Review the "Cardiovascular Training Guidelines" near the end of this chapter for additional help in designing your program.

EXERCISE PLAN #3 - FLEXIBILITY / STRETCHING EXERCISES

After your aerobics training three days a week, you should conduct The Healthy

Aging Stretching Workout. Review the "Flexibility Exercise Guidelines" near the end of this chapter, paying particular attention to the five key points to maximize the workout. The entire upper and lower body program can be conducted in five to 10 minutes after you become familiar with the 10 different recommended stretches.

EXERCISE PLAN #3 - STRENGTH TRAINING

Train three days a week using either weight machines, free weights or resistance training. Always warm up prior to any strength training routine. If you did not participate in Exercise Plan #2, review "How to Estimate 80 Percent of Your One Repetition Maximum (80% 1RM)" on page 58, and the more detailed explanation at the end of this chapter.

Alternate your schedule each week as follows:

Week 1: Upper Body, Lower Body, Upper Body
Week 2: Lower Body, Upper Body, Lower Body

Upper Body: Back, Chest, Shoulders, Bicep and Triceps
Choose two exercises for each of the upper body parts listed and complete the following: three sets of 10 repetitions at 80% 1RM for each body part.

Lower Body: Quadriceps, Hamstrings, Calves and Abdominals
Choose 2 exercises for each of the lower body parts listed and complete the following: three sets of 10 repetitions at 80% 1RM for each body part.

Review the "Strength Training Guidelines" near the end of this chapter for help in designing your own program.

SUMMARY: HEALTHY AGING EXERCISE PLAN #3
Following is a typical Exercise Plan #3 weekly schedule. In this example, the upper body is getting exercised two times. Be sure, on the following week, to switch and exercise the lower body two times. Flexibility/stretching exercises should be done on the cardiovascular days, after your aerobic workout. Notice that with Plan #3, you will increase the intensity of the strength training exercises to three sets of 10 repetitions each at 80 percent of 1RM, instead of three sets of 6-8 repetitions as in Exercise Plan #2.

EXERCISE PLAN #3 WEEKLY GUIDE

Monday	Upper Body Strength Training
Tuesday	25 Minutes of Aerobics plus Flexibility/Stretching Exercises
Wednesday	Lower Body Strength Training
Thursday	25 Minutes of Interval Aerobics plus Flexibility/Stretching Exercises
Friday	Upper Body Strength Training
Saturday	25 minutes of Aerobics plus Flexibility/Stretching Exercises
Sunday	Rest

CARDIOVASCULAR TRAINING GUIDELINES

WHAT EXERCISES SHOULD I DO?

There are many activities that can improve your aerobic fitness. Walking is one of the best overall activities. Walking can be done almost anywhere, and it requires no special equipment to purchase. Walking puts very little strain on your joints and involves all the major muscle groups. It can be done alone or with a group at various paces that are comfortable.

WALKING THE RIGHT WAY

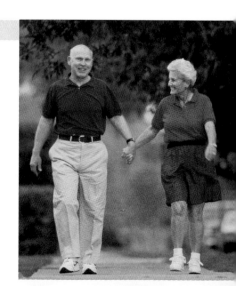

One of the biggest mistakes walkers make is bending forward, which leads to problems in your lower back, neck and hips. You should walk naturally tall. You don't need to force yourself to be ramrod straight, nor should you slouch over. Relax your shoulders, widen your chest and pull your abdominals gently inward. Keep your head and chin up and focus straight ahead. Keep your hands relaxed and cupped gently and swing your arms so that they just brush past your body. On the upswing, your hand should be level with your breastbone. On the downswing, you hand should brush against your hip. Keep your hips loose and relaxed. Your feet should land firmly with your heels first. Roll through your heel to your arch, then to the ball of your foot and then finally to your toes. Push off from your toes and the ball of your foot.

TIPS FOR WALKING

Even though walking is the most basic of all fitness activities, here are some key points for success:

• WALK AS FAST AS YOU CAN...COMFORTABLY!

Over time, gradually increase your workout time and pace. If you walk at a 12-minute mile to a 15-minute mile pace, you will burn twice as many calories as when you walk at a 20-minute mile pace. You may not be able to walk at such a fast pace in the beginning, but as you get more fit, you can mix in some fast-paced intervals, using the 25-minute Interval Aerobics Workout as a guide.

• CONQUER SOME HILLS

Walking up hills or over hilly terrain will help shape your buttocks and thighs and actually burns about 30 percent more calories than walking on flat terrain.

• WALK WHENEVER YOU CAN

Think about leaving your car at home for a change and walk to the store. Take a 15-minute walk during your lunch break. Walk up more stairs instead of using the elevator. Anytime and anywhere you can, sneak in some extra walking.

RUNNING THE RIGHT WAY

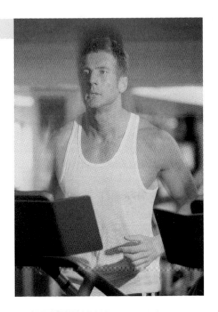

Running is an excellent way to get into cardiovascular shape. But make certain you gradually work up to running. If you are new to the fitness game, start out slowly.

Some runners seem to have the habit of looking directly at the ground as they run. Keeping your head down will throw off your upper body posture and may lead to neck and upper back pain. Lift your head up and focus your eyes straight ahead. Relax your shoulders; keep your chest lifted up. Pull in your abdominal muscles. Be careful not to over arch your back or stick your buttocks out. This is one of the main reasons that runners get back and hip pain.

Keep your arms close to your body and swing them forward and back rather than across your body. Keep your fists relaxed, and don't clench them. Visualize that you are holding a small bird in your hand. You don't want to crush it, nor do you want the bird to fly off.

Lift your front knee and extend your back leg. Be careful not to shuffle along like you are wearing heavy boots. Land your heel first and roll through the entire length of your foot. Push off from the balls of your feet instead of running flat-footed and pounding your heels. If you don't follow these tips, you may feel pain in your feet and legs. If you feel pain in your ankles, knees or lower back, stop running for a while, then start over "running the right way."

TIPS FOR RUNNING
The following tips will help you become fit and avoid possible injuries.

• BEGIN BY ALTERNATING WALKING WITH RUNNING
As an example, try about two minutes of walking and one minute of running. Then you can gradually increase your running intervals until you can comfortably run continuously for 20 minutes.

• CHANGE YOUR PACE
If you run at different paces, you will work your heart, lungs and your legs in various ways. Mix it up a bit and experiment with several techniques that work for you.

• BE CAREFUL NOT TO INCREASE YOUR MILEAGE MORE THAN 10 PERCENT PER WEEK
For example you have worked up to five miles per week, and you want to increase your mileage, focus on increasing to about 5.5 miles the following week. If you drastically increase from five to six miles, studies indicate that you may set yourself up for injury.

• DON'T RUN EVERY DAY
We recommend that you rest at least one day per week. We also suggest that you might want to alternate running with other activities that may be less jarring on your joints, such as swimming or cycling, or you can refer to the list on page 62

WHAT ACTIVITIES BURN THE MOST CALORIES?

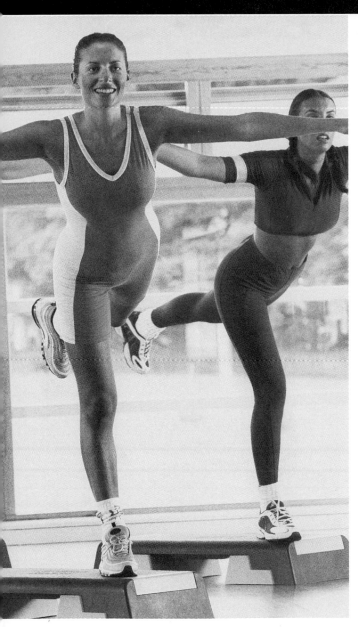

The following list gives calorie estimates for a number of favorite aerobic activities. The number of calories that you actually burn will depend upon the intensity of your workout, your weight, your muscle mass and your metabolism. As an example, a beginner will burn approximately 4 or 5 calories per minute of exercise, while once you become fit, you will burn 10 to 12 calories per minute.

We have included several sports in which your activity level is not constant, such as basketball and tennis. These activities are not "truly aerobic," but they can still give you a great workout and add to your overall program for weight loss and increased well-being.

The number of calories burned in this list is for a person who weighs 150 pounds.

LIST OF CALORIES BURNED PER ACTIVITY

ACTIVITY	15 MIN	30 MIN	45 MIN	60 MIN
• Aerobic Dance	171	342	513	684
• Basketball	141	282	432	564
• Bicycling				
12 mph	142	283	425	566
15 mph	177	354	531	708
18 mph	213	425	638	850
• Cross-country Skiing	146	291	437	583
• Downhill Skiing	105	210	315	420
• Golf (carrying clubs)	87	174	261	348
• In-line Skating	150	300	450	600
• Jumping Rope				
60-80 skips per min.	143	286	429	572
• Karate, Tae Kwon Do	192	834	576	768
• Kayaking	75	150	225	300
• Racquetball	114	228	342	456
• Rowing Machine	104	208	310	415
• Running				
10-minute mile	183	365	548	731
8-minute mile	223	446	670	893
• Ski Machine	141	282	423	564
• Swimming				
Freestyle-35 yds/min.	124	248	371	497
Freestyle-50 yds/min.	131	261	392	523

- **Tennis**

Singles	116	232	348	464
Doubles	43	85	128	170

- **Versa Climber**

100 ft./min	188	375	563	750

- **Walking**

20-minute mile Flat	60	120	180	240
20-minute mile Hills	81	162	243	324
15-minute mile Flat	73	146	219	292
15-minute mile Hills	102	206	279	412

- **Water Aerobics**

	70	140	210	280

Remember, getting into good cardiovascular shape is an important "ongoing" life project. You might have to struggle a bit through the first sessions, but if you stick with it three times per week for at least six weeks, you will start to notice dramatic changes. After a few weeks, you will recover much more quickly from your workouts. After your workout, instead of crashing on the couch, you will start to feel energized, handle stress, look better and improve your overall vitality.

FLEXIBILITY / STRETCHING EXERCISE GUIDELINES

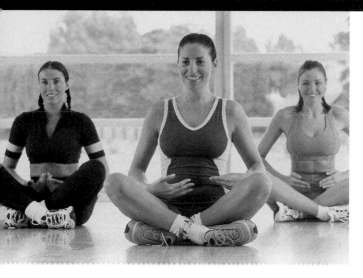

This section will provide an easy stretching workout that focuses on classic stretches. Once you become familiar with these moves, the workout should take you only about five minutes. Here are a few key points to maximize your stretching workout:

- **Stretch on a regular basis-daily, if you can:** Always stretch after every work-out, whether you are doing cardiovascular work or strength training. When you stretch on the days that you don't work out, be careful to warm up properly with a few minutes of easy movement like shoulder rolls, gentle waist twists or light cardio activity.

- **Gently move into each stretching position:** Never force yourself into a stretch by jerking or snapping into position.

- **Be aware of how much tension you feel:** When you stretch properly, you should rate anywhere from mild tension to the edge of discomfort on your "pain meter." It should never cause severe or sharp pain anywhere else in your body. Focus on the area that you are stretching and notice the stretch spread through these muscles.

- **Hold each stretch for 10 slow counts:** When you find a comfortable stretch position, stay there or gradually deepen the stretch. Don't bounce! Bouncing only serves to tighten your muscles, not loosen them. Forceful bouncing increases the risk of tearing a muscle.

- **Take two deep breaths as you hold each position:** Deep breathing will promote relaxation and provides a shot of oxygen into your muscles.

STRETCHING ROUTINE

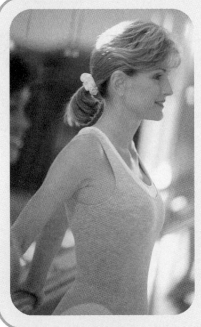

NECK STRETCH

This stretch is designed to relax and loosen up the muscles in your neck.

Sit or stand comfortably. Drop your left ear toward your left shoulder. Gently stretch your right arm down and a few inches out to the side. Repeat the stretch on your right side.

REMEMBER:
- Keep your shoulders down and relaxed.
- Your ear may or may not touch your shoulder, depending how flexible you are.

CHEST EXPANSION

This move targets your shoulders, chest and arms and also helps promote good posture.

Sit or stand up tall and bring your arms behind you, clasping one hand inside the other. Lift your chest and raise your arms slightly. You should feel a mild stretch spread across your chest and down the back of your arms.

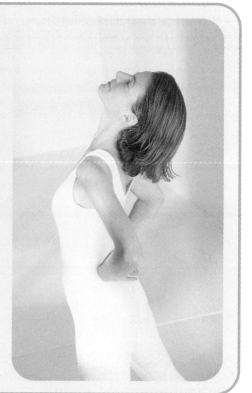

REMEMBER:
- Try to keep your shoulders relaxed and down.
- Resist arching your lower back as you pull your arms upward.
- Don't force your arms up higher than is comfortable.

BACK EXPANSION

This stretches and loosens your shoulders, arms, upper back and lower back muscles.

Standing tall with your knees slightly bent and feet hip-width apart, lift your arms in front of you to shoulder height. Clasp one hand in the other. Drop your head toward your chest, pull your abdominals inward, round your lower back and tuck your hips forward so that you create a "C" shape with your torso. Stretch your arms forward so that you feel your shoulder blades gently moving apart and you create an "opposition" to your rounded back. You should feel a mild stretch slowly spread through your back, shoulders and arms.

REMEMBER:
- Keep your abdominal muscles pulled inward to protect your lower back.
- Keep your shoulders down and relaxed.
- Lean only as far forward as you feel comfortable and balanced.

STANDING HAMSTRING STRETCH

This move is a great stretch for your hamstrings or rear thigh muscles, as well as your lower back. If you have lower back problems, do the same exercise while lying on your back on the floor and extending your leg upward.

Stand tall with your left foot a few inches in front of your right foot and your left toes lifted. Bend your right knee slightly and pull your abdominals gently inward. Lean forward from your hips and rest both palms on top of your right thigh for balance and support. Keep your shoulders down and relaxed and don't round your back. You should feel a mild pull gradually spread through the back of your leg. Repeat the stretch with your right leg forward.

 REMEMBER:
• Don't lean so far forward that you lose your balance or feel strain in your lower back.
• Keep your back straight and your abs pulled inward to make the stretch more effective and to protect your lower back.

STANDING QUAD STRETCH

This stretch really concentrates on the quadriceps or front thigh muscles. Be very careful to move gently with this stretch, especially if you are prone to knee or lower back pain. If you are experiencing back pain, you can do a similar stretch while lying on your side, bending your top knee and bringing your heel toward your buttocks.

Stand tall with your feet hip-width apart, pull your abdominals in, and relax your shoulders. Bend your left leg, bringing your heel toward your buttocks and grasp your left foot with your right hand. You should begin to feel a mild pull gradually spread through the front of your left leg. Then repeat legs.

 REMEMBER:
• Don't lock the knee of your base leg.
• Hold on to a chair or the wall if you have trouble balancing.

DOUBLE CALF STRETCH

This move can give you some real relief for tight and bunched-up calf muscles that may result from daily activities such as walking and standing.

Stand with your feet together about 2 feet from a wall that you are facing. Pull your abs gently inward and don't round your lower back. With straight arms, press your palms into the wall and lean forward from your ankles, keeping your heels pressed as close to the floor as possible. You should feel a mild stretch spread through your calf muscles.

REMEMBER:
- Keep your abs pulled in to prevent your lower back from sagging or arching.
- Keep both heels flat on the floor or as close to the floor as your flexibility allows.
- To increase the stretch, bend your elbows, leaning your chest towards the wall.

SUN SALUTATION

This stretch will focus on your abs, lower back, front hip and thigh muscles. If you are prone to lower back pain, make a special point of tightening your abs, and don't arch your lower back.

Kneel on the floor and then bring your left leg forward so that your foot is flat on the floor with your knees bent and your thigh is parallel to the floor. Lift your arms straight up with your palms facing inward. Pull your abs gently inward, and keep your shoulders down and back. Look to the ceiling and as you stretch upward with your upper body, push your weight slightly forward from your hips into your front thigh. You will begin to feel this stretch travel through your torso and upper body, including your arms. You should also feel it at the very top of your back thigh. Repeat with your right leg forward.

REMEMBER:
- Hold onto something solid, such as a sturdy chair, with one hand if you have trouble maintaining your balance.
- Don't lean so far forward that your front knee moves in front of your toes.
- Don't arch your lower back.

HORSE BITING TAIL

This stretch may have an odd name, but it is great for stretching your abdominals, sides and lower back. Be careful not to force this stretch, particularly if you have lower back problems.

Kneel on your hands and knees so that your palms are directly beneath your shoulders. Your knees should be directly below your hips. Pull your abs gently inward so that your back neither sags nor arches. Slowly twist your spine to the left as much as your flexibility allows, so that you are looking back over your shoulder toward your left buttock and your left buttock moves slightly forward. You should feel a mild stretch spread through your spine. Slowly move back to center and repeat to the right.

REMEMBER:
- Keep your abs pulled in to prevent your lower back from sagging.
- Don't force the stretch.

BUTTERFLY STRETCH

This move will stretch your inner thighs, groin, hips and lower back. If you are prone to lower back problems, take extra care to lean forward from your hips rather than rounding your lower back. This exercise may also cause some knee discomfort.

Sit up tall with the soles of your feet pressed together and your knees dropped to the sides as far as they will comfortably go. Pull your abs gently inward and lean forward from your hips. Grasp your feet with your hands and carefully pull yourself a small way further forward. You should feel the stretch spread throughout your inner thighs the outermost part of your hips, as well as in your lower back.

REMEMBER:
- Don't hunch your shoulders up toward your ears or round your back.
- Increase the stretch by carefully pressing your thighs toward the floor as you hold the position.
- To reduce stress on your knees, move your feet away from your body.
- To increase the stretch, move your feet toward your body.

CHILD'S POSE

This move will stretch your lower back and arms and relaxes your entire body. If you have knee problems, lower yourself into the position with extra care.

Start in a kneeling position. Drop your buttocks toward your heels as you stretch the rest of your body down and forward. In the fully stretched position, your arms should be resting in a relaxed position along the floor, your stomach should be resting comfortably on top of your thighs, and your forehead should be resting on a mat or the floor. You will begin to feel a mild stretch in your shoulders and buttocks and down the length of your spine and arms.

REMEMBER:
- Ease into this stretch by keeping your shoulders and neck relaxed.
- Don't force your buttocks to move any closer to your heels than is comfortable.

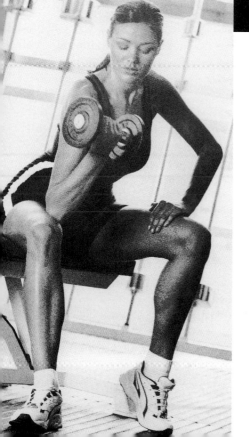

STRENGTH TRAINING GUIDELINES

Scientists at world-renowned research institutions agree that a decline in muscle strength and size is not inevitable as we age. Landmark research at a university in Boston, Mass., disproved the conventional thinking that age somehow decreases the ability of the muscles to get bigger in response to strength training, a belief firmly held by most lay people and still referenced in many scientific journals.

Early researchers in many strength-building studies went wrong, according to the director of this research, because they did not push their older subjects hard enough. The researchers assumed their older subjects couldn't withstand anything beyond very low-intensity training. Usually this meant 30 to 40 percent of their maximal lifting capacity.

Exercise physiologists know to improve strength in young people to any worthwhile degree, they must lift between 60 and 100 percent of their maximal capacity.

This study had older subjects, ages 60 to 72, train at 80 percent of their one repetition maximum (1RM), or 80 percent of the most weight they could lift with one try.

The subjects trained three days a week for 12 weeks. Since the subjects were getting stronger all the time, the weight had to be adjusted upward every week to have them continue to lift 80 percent of their 1RM.

The results of the study, tested by CT scan and muscle biopsy, made healthcare providers revise their thinking about strength building among senior citizens. The individuals in the research program had their quadriceps (front of thigh) muscle strength increase by more than 200 percent and their hamstring (back of thigh) muscle strength by 300 percent!

The conclusion of the study was that indeed, hypertrophy or muscle growth had occurred, and the amount of hypertrophy was as much as could be expected from young people doing the same amount of exercise.

YOUR ONE REPETITION MAXIMUM (1RM)

First, you must familiarize yourself with the term one repetition maximum (1RM). This is the most weight you can lift with one try. If you try lifting that amount of weight again immediately afterward, you can't, because your muscles are too tired.

Clearly, your 1RM is like a fingerprint. It's unique to you. Once you have accurately estimated your 1RM, you will be asked to lift, as part of your Healthy Aging Program, about 80 percent of your 1RM amount. For example if the most weight you can bench press one time is 50 pounds, you would use 80 percent of this amount or 40 pounds.

However, over the weeks of the program, you'll find that your 1RM, the heaviest weight you can lift at any given time, changes. As your muscles grow bigger and stronger, you'll be able to substitute heavier and heavier weights. That's why the Healthy Aging Program is a progressive, resistance-training program for life.

Unfortunately, 80 percent of your 1RM is difficult to measure unless you have a large selection of weights to choose from and a professional at your side, helping guide your lifts. A general guideline to estimate 80 percent of your 1RM on a continuous basis is as follows.

HOW TO ESTIMATE 80 PERCENT OF YOUR ONE REPETITION MAXIMUM (80% 1RM)

When doing a bench press, if you can lift the weight more than twelve times, it's too light or below 80 percent of your 1RM. If, on the other hand, you can only lift the weight eight times or less, it's too heavy or higher than 80 percent of your 1RM. The ideal estimate of 80% 1RM would have you lifting the weight between 9 to 10 repetitions, with repetition eight being difficult, repetition nine being very difficult, and repetition 10 creating failure.

THE NUMBER OF STRENGTH TRAINING SETS AND REPETITIONS

In our Healthy Aging Weight Training (or resistance exercise) Program you will typically be performing three sets of each exercise, with each set consisting of 10 repetitions. The set and repetition amount won't change throughout the course of the program. What will change is the intensity or amount of weight that you will lift.

Every week you should be aware of your lifting ability, and adjust upward the weight amount if you exceed 10 repetitions for any exercise.

You must alternate your weight training and/or resistance exercises between upper and lower body every other workout. For example, one week on Monday and Friday do upper body exercises and lower body exercises on Wednesday. The following week do lower body exercises on Monday and Friday and upper body exercises on Wednesday.

When doing your upper body, perform two exercises per body part exercised, conducting three sets of 10 repetitions. Chest, shoulders, triceps, biceps and back should be exercised on each upper body day and quadriceps, hamstrings, calves and abdominals on each lower body day. By striving to rest only 60 seconds between sets, the entire upper or lower body program will take less than 45 minutes.

In addition, your healthcare provider who put you on the Healthy Aging program will regularly reevaluate your health and fitness level by conducting a follow up *Actual*Age™ Assessment and comparing it to your last test.

WHAT KIND OF STRENGTH TRAINING SHOULD I DO?

The following section of this book details the different kinds of strength training available: weight machines, free weights and iron-free resistance training. There are a variety of exercises described for each of the three types of strength training.

Vary from week to week the type of exercise conducted for each body part to prevent the body from adapting to any one particular exercise.

Building muscle is very important, no matter which method or equipment that you choose to use.

WHICHEVER METHOD YOU CHOOSE, REMEMBER THESE IMPORTANT FITNESS TIPS:

- Always warm up before you exercise.
- Make sure you work each muscle or muscle group to fatigue.
- Start with light weights.
- Continue to challenge your muscles by increasing the weights and making your workout a bit harder as you get stronger.
- You can challenge yourself by several methods: increasing reps, increasing sets, increasing weight or decreasing resting time.
- Perform your strength training every other day. Give your body a day to rest and recover after each workout.
- Do gentle stretching after each workout.

WEIGHT MACHINES

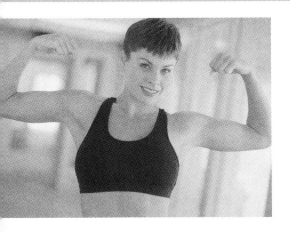

You can find most weight machines in your local gyms or clubs. There are generally several machines to work on specific muscle groups, as well as a common weight apparatus typically called a multi-station machine. These machines will work on: shoulders, back, chest, biceps, triceps, outer and inner thighs, hamstrings and quadriceps.

The following chart outlines 10 great exercises for typical weight machines. Remember, no two brands of weight machines are alike. Therefore, we recommend you work with a trainer or weight-room attendant who can properly introduce you to the machines.

TEN GREAT WEIGHT MACHINES

1)   • Machine: **CHEST FLY**

• Muscle Group: Pectorals (Chest)

• Result:

 - Men: sculpted chest

 - Women: firmer and sometimes larger breasts

• Performance Position:
 While seated, raise your forearms to chest level, place them behind padded panels or grip handles, and press them together in front of you. On other machines, you might lie on your back and grasp handles above your chest, extend your arms out to your sides, and bring them up above your chest. Return to the starting position.

2)   • Machine: **CHEST PRESS**

• Muscle Group: Pectorals (Chest)

• Result:

 - Men: sculpted chest

 - Women: firmer and sometimes larger breasts

• Performance Position:
 While seated, grasp the handles in front of you at chest level and push them away from your body. Bend your elbows to return to the starting position.

3)   • Machine: **SHOULDER PRESS**

      • Muscle Group: Deltoids (Shoulders)

      • Result:
        Well-developed shoulders that make your waist
        look narrower

      • Performance Position:
        While seated, grasp the handles at chest or
        shoulder level and push them straight up. For some
        machines, sit leaning forward slightly.
        Lower your arms to return to the starting position.

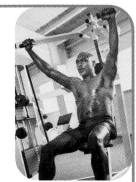

4)   • Machine: **UPRIGHT ROW**

      • Muscle Group: Trapezius, Deltoids, Rhomboids and Biceps
        (Shoulders and Upper Arms)

      • Result:
        Broad shoulders that make your waist appear narrower

      • Performance Position:
        Stand with your arms extended in front of your hips, grasp the
        handles. Bending and raising the elbows, pull them back and up to
        shoulder level. Lower your arms to return to the starting position.

5)   • Machine: **ARM OR BICEPS CURL**

      • Muscle Group: Biceps (Front of upper arms)

      • Result:
        Defined biceps, one of the classic muscles that
        indicates muscle mass

      • Performance Position:
        While seated with your arms in front of you, grasp the handles and
        pull them up toward your chest, bending at the elbows. Straighten
        your elbows to return to the starting position.

6) • Machine: **TRICEPS PRESS**

     • Muscle Group: Triceps (Back of upper arms)

     • Result:
Toned triceps that eliminate flabby upper
arms, especially in women.

     • Performance Position:
While seated, grasp the handles at your sides with your elbows bent
and straighten your arms, pressing downward and back. Bend your
elbows and return to the starting position.

7) • Machine: **SEATED ROW**

     • Muscle Group: Latissimi dorsi, Trapezius,
Rhomboids, Biceps and Erector Spine (Back)

     • Result:
Strong back for pulling, lifting, standing
and sitting erect. Overall good posture.

     • Performance Position:
While seated with your legs bent, grasp the handles
in front of you and pull them back, bending the elbows,
like you are rowing a boat. Return to the starting position.

8) • Machine: **LAT-PULL DOWN**

     • Muscle Group: Latissimi dorsi (Back)

     • Result:
Defined lats that help make your hips look
narrower

     • Performance Position:
While seated, grasp the overhead bar and pull it
down in front of your body to chest level, leaning back slightly. The
weights will pull your arms upward to return to the starting position.

9).   • Machine: **LEG PRESS**

   • Muscle Group: Quadriceps and Gluteals (Front of thighs and buttocks)

   • Result:
   Firm and toned lower body

   • Performance Position:
   While lying on your back with your knees bent, place your feet against
   a pad and push your legs forward and up, stopping a few degrees short
   of straightening your legs. Bend your knees back toward your chest to
   return to the starting position.

10).   • Machine: **LEG CURL**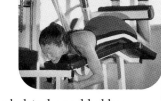

   • Muscle Group: Hamstrings (Back of thighs)

   • Result:
   A firm and shapely behind

   • Performance Position:
   Lying: While lying face down, hook your ankles behind a padded bar,
   press your hips down, and bend your knees to bring your heels up
   toward your buttocks. Straighten your legs to return to the starting
   position.

FREE WEIGHTS

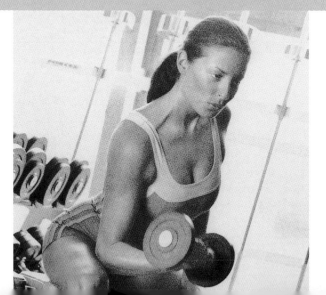

As part of your strength-training program, you may wish to use barbells or free weights. If you are a beginner, light dumbbells are the free weights that you want to use. These weights generally start with one-pounders and then increase in small increments from there. The typical weight increments in pounds are as follows: 1, 2, 3, 5, 8, 10, 12.5, 15, 17.5, 20 and 22.5. There are even some weights that are more, e.g. up to 50 pounds.

In general, you want to hold the weights lightly, but firmly, in your hands without clutching them too hard. We recommend that you start with light weights and gradually progress to heavier ones. There are many variations for dumbbell exercises. Following are six great free-weight exercises:

1. ARM/BICEPS CURL: You can also do these curls while sitting on a bench or standing with your feet about shoulder-width apart. Bend your knees slightly and put your arms straight down and close to your body. Bend your elbows up to your chest. Straighten your arms and lower the weights to the starting position. The term "arm curl" or "biceps curl" is used when you do this exercise with the palms facing toward the ceiling. When you rotate your forearms so that your thumbs are facing the ceiling, then this is called a "hammer curl." When you perform the exercise with palms facing the floor, it is called a "reverse curl." Each one of these variations strengthens the biceps and the muscles of the forearms in slightly different ways.

2. FORWARD ARM RAISE: Stand with your feet about shoulder-width apart, or you can also sit on a bench. Keep your left arm at your side and raise your right arm straight in front of you to shoulder height. Then alternate bringing your left arm up and your right arm down. Then bring your right arm up and your left arm down. This exercise strengthens your shoulder muscles.

3. TRICEPS CURL: This exercise can be performed with one weight in each hand or with a heavier weight held in both hands. Stand with your feet about shoulder width apart, or you can sit on a bench. Raise your arms straight overhead, keeping them close to your ears, and bend your elbows, lowering the weights behind you. Straighten your arms to raise the weights to the starting position.

4. LATERAL RAISE: Stand with your feet about shoulder-width apart. Have your palms facing each other, raise both arms out to your sides to ear level. Return to the starting position. This exercise strengthens the shoulders, specifically focusing on the deltoids.

5. CHEST PRESS: Lie on your back on a mat or bench with your elbows bent, your hands at chest level, and your palms toward your feet. Press your hands upward and straighten your elbows without locking them. Bend them to return to the starting position. This exercise strengthens the shoulders, triceps and pectorals. You can also perform this exercise with a barbell held by both hands. When you do it on a bench, which gives you greater range of motion, it is called a "bench press."

6. FLY: Lie on your back on a bench with your elbows slightly bent and your hands above your chest. If you are not comfortable on a bench, you also can do this exercise lying on a mat. You won't experience as much range of motion, but it is a variation you could try. Extend your arms out to the side. Alternately open them and bring them together above your chest. This exercise will strengthen your chest.

LEG WEIGHTS

The most popular leg weights are ones that wrap around your leg with flexible, padded Velcro closures. Some designs feature lead-bar weights that slip into pouches that can be adjusted for weight as well as size. Other designs such as Lei Weights contain small heavy pellets. This design is soft and comfortable and can be draped over the leg or used in place of dumbbells in other free weight exercises. No matter which design you prefer, here are two of the most common lower body exercises that use leg weights:

1. INNER-THIGH LEG LIFT: Lie on your left side with your hip bones stacked one above the other, perpendicular to the floor, with your left knee slightly bent. Bend your top leg and place it on the floor in front of your body. Raise your bottom leg off the floor and lower it to the starting position. Be sure to lift your leg without rolling onto your buttock. Switch to the other side. Your goal should be the same number of reps and sets on each side as for the outer-thigh leg lift. This exercise tones the inner thighs.

2. OUTER-THIGH LEG LIFT: Lie on your left side with your hip bones stacked one above the other, perpendicular to the floor, with your left knee slightly bent. Lift your right leg up and down. You can lift it and alternately bend and extend the knee, or you can combine these movements so that on each rep you lift, extend, bend, and lower your leg. Switch to the other side. This exercise tones your outer thighs.

There are many weight-training accessories for specific situations. If you have arthritis and gripping hand weights is uncomfortable, you can experiment with the heavy-duty plastic extenders called EZ Grips. These extenders will provide a larger, more comfortable surface to hold. Some people use support belts to prevent abdominal and back injuries while lifting weights. Still others prefer wearing gloves while working with weights to avoid blisters and to protect the hands. These products are available at stores that sell specialized exercise equipment.

IRON-FREE RESISTANCE TRAINING

(Pumping Your Body Instead of Iron)

Some of these exercises, such as push ups and abdominal crunches, require that you lift your own body weight. Other exercises are traditional calisthenics that you might have done in a gym class in high school. These exercises get joints and muscles moving, which provide general toning and mobility conditioning.

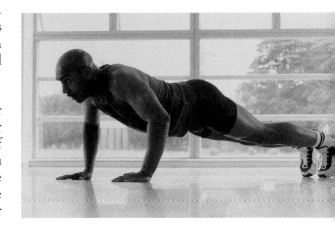

Exercises that rely on your body instead of other gear have the added benefit of "portability." Wherever you go, you can perform these exercises, whether you have a job that requires travel or you are on a camping trip.

ABDOMINAL CRUNCHES

The commonly used word "abdominals" includes the rectus abdominus, a flat wedged-shaped muscle reaching from the rib cage to the pubic bone; the obliques, which are on each side of the waist and the transverse abdominus, which wraps around the waist like a cummerbund.

Ab crunches are one of the most basic abdominal exercises in fitness. There are many variations of this exercise. In all of them, you begin by lying on your back with your lower back pressed against the mat or floor. Bend your knees and put your feet flat on the floor. Begin by contracting the abdominal muscles and then slowly lift and lower your head, shoulders and upper back.

You can select your arm position. If you feel tension in your neck region, place your hands behind your head with your fingers interlaced or touching. If your

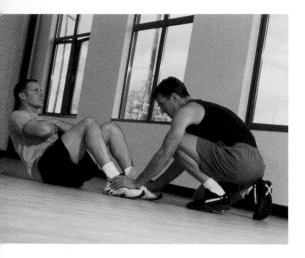

neck does not bother you, you can extend your arms straight in front of you or overhead. You can also place them on your thighs and slide them up as you lift your upper body, shoulders and head. If you are comfortable in doing so, you can cross your hands over your chest.

If you raise your feet slightly off the floor, which releases the weight from them as you lift your upper body, it makes the crunches more challenging.

Protect your back by tilting your pelvis forward so your entire spine is in contact with the floor and contract your abdominals to keep it that way. To work deeper into the lower section of your abs, or the rectus abdominus, keep your heels on the floor, but alternately raise your left toes and then your right toes as you come up for each crunch.

Whatever position you prefer, keep your tummy tight so that your lower back presses against the mat or the floor. You can visualize pressing your bellybutton through your back to the floor. Work through the entire exercise slowly and steadily, without heaving yourself up or flopping down.

MODIFIED CRUNCHES

Crunches work the entire rectus abdominus area, but several other exercises also focus on the lower section of the abs. The easiest of these is a crunch with a bit of a change.

Lie on your back as you would to start your regular crunches, but let your knees fall outward, keeping your feet together. When you do your crunches from this butterfly position, you will feel your lower abs handling much more of the load.

To tone the "love handle" area on the sides of your body, you need to work

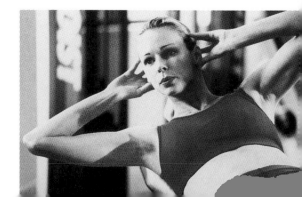

on your obliques. One of the best versions is to place your hands behind your head for support and begin alternating your left shoulder toward your right knee, and then your right shoulder toward your left knee.

You can increase the intensity of your abdominal exercises by doing a "pulse set" after your regular crunches. Pressing your lower back to the mat or floor, pulse for one set at the top of the exercise and then hold the very highest position for a count of 10. Remember to breathe.

Other advanced ab work includes more challenging positions. You can lift your legs off the floor and cross your ankles when you do your crunches to really work your waist. Reverse curls are the power exercise for the lower abs. Lie on your back, lift your legs straight up or raise them and cross them at your ankles, and place your hands under your pelvis to support your back. Contract your abdominals to raise your hips off the floor. Be certain to tighten your tummy with each lift; otherwise, your back and hip flexor will do most of the work. Then when your abs are really strong, you can further intensify your exercises by combining crunches and reverse curls.

After you work your abs, remain on your back to stretch out. First, raise your hands above your head and stretch your arms, legs and torso, elongating your entire body. Next, bring your knees up to a bent position and let them fall to one side of your body. Stretch your arms to the other side. You can also roll over onto your abdomen with your legs stretched behind you. Place your hands, palms down, on either side of your body and raise your upper body. Stop at a comfortable point to protect your back.

PUSH-UPS
If you are inexperienced with push-ups, always start very gently and modestly. Get down on your hands and knees on the floor or on a mat.

Full or "Military" Push-Ups
These are the most difficult version of this exercise. Keep your body straight, supporting your weight on your hands and toes. Begin bending and straightening your elbows to raise and lower your body. You can do full push-ups to fatigue and then complete the exercise set with the easier version, if you wish.

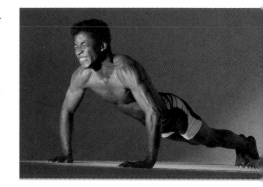

"Girl" Push-Ups

This level of push up has this nick-name because even many fit women who cannot build upper body strength like men do them. Start with your feet and shins on the floor and your hands a little more than shoul-der-width apart. Keeping your back straight, bend your elbows to lower your shoulders and upper body until your fore-head and nose almost touch the floor. Straighten your elbows to raise yourself. You can begin with two sets of eight or 10 push-ups, and when you are comfort-able doing these, continue until you cannot complete one more fully.

Wall Push-Ups

You can even ease into push-ups by starting from a standing position and hold-ing on to a horizontal support such as a sturdy deck railing or ballet bar. Bend your elbows to angle your upper body toward the support and straighten them to return to the starting position.

Stretching After Push-Ups

Proper stretching after you complete this exercise will help relax your arms, shoulders and back. First, stay in the kneeling position with your feet flattened against the floor. Shift your hips back until you are sitting on your lower legs. Stretch your arms in front of you. Then, sit with your legs crossed comfortably in front of you and reach behind your back, clasp your hands together, and press them back to stretch your upper arms, shoulders and chest. Then bring your hands in front of your body, clasp them at shoulder level, and round your back to stretch your arms, shoulders and upper back.

TRICEPS DIPS

Sit at the edge of a sturdy straight chair or weight bench with your feet slightly in front of you and slightly apart. Place your hands on the edge of the seat next to your hips with your palms down and your fingers forward. Slide off the seat, supporting your weight on your hands. Bend your elbows 90 degrees, flexing your knees to lower your hips toward the floor. Then straighten your elbows to return to the starting position with your hips level with the seat. Slide back onto the seat to rest between sets or whenever you need to.

To stretch, raise your right arm and bend it behind your head. Grasp your right elbow with your left hand and press back against your forearm with the back of your head. Switch sides.

LEG LIFTS

Lie on your right side with your hips stacked. You might want to prop your head on your right hand to be more comfortable, or you might prefer to extend your right arm out and cushion your head on it. To work your outer thigh, bend your right leg to a 45-degree angle from your body for stability. Raise your left leg from the hip until it is parallel to the floor and then lower it to the starting position. When you are ready for a slightly more advanced exercise, straighten your knee while your leg is raised, bend it, straighten it, and then lower it. When you can easily do two or three sets of each of these, you can add a set of small pulses and hold your leg up at the highest part of the lift for a count of eight and release. Switch to the other side.

To work your inner thighs, lie on your right side with your hips stacked. Cross your left leg over your right and place your left foot on the floor. This moves it out of the way of the right leg, which will be your working leg for this exercise. Lift and lower your right leg. When you are strong enough, finish with small pulses and then contract your muscles to hold your working leg at the highest part of the lift for a count of eight and then release. Switch legs.

REAR LEG LIFTS

To work your hamstrings and gluteals, get down on all fours on a mat or on the floor. To protect your back, lower your elbows so that your forearms are resting on the floor. Raise and lower your right leg, keeping it straight behind you and elevating it no higher than the level of your hips. Then bend your right knee and raise and lower your leg with your foot flexed and the sole pointing to the ceiling. You can add a set of pulses in each position, and when you are stronger, you can finish by holding your leg up for a count of eight to 15 seconds. Another variation is to raise your leg with your knee straight, then bend it so that the sole of your foot points at the ceiling, straighten it again, and then lower it. Repeat with the left leg.

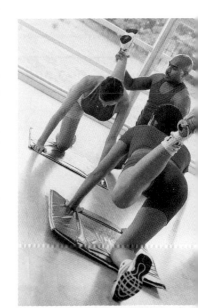

GLUTEAL SQUEEZE

To tone your buttocks, lie on your back on a mat or on the floor with your feet shoulder-width apart. Keep your lower back pressed to the floor and raise your hips, and then alternately squeeze and release your gluteal muscles. This is a very small motion. By keeping your feet in place but bringing your knees together, or by moving your feet a few inches farther apart or closer together, you will vary the exercise slightly and work a slightly different area. Finish the exercise by contracting the muscles as hard as you can and holding for eight to 15 seconds.

SQUATS

If you don't have knee problems, this is a tried-and-true lower body exercise. It helps strengthen and tone the quadriceps, hamstrings, calves and glutes. Stand with your toes pointing straight ahead and your feet hip-width apart. Keep a natural posture with your back straight. Keep your knees pointing straight ahead and press your hips forward, keeping your back straight and without bending at the waist. You can steady yourself with a chair back, a bar or another support if you need to, or you can rest your hands on your thighs or keep them out in front of you for balance.

Keeping your feet firmly on the floor and your heels pressed down, squat slowly and no deeper than 90 degrees, which is no lower than a position in which your thighs are parallel to the floor. Rise up at the same tempo, pushing your body back to a standing position. When you get stronger, you can add extra weight in the form of dumbbells at your sides, or even a barbell across your shoulders.

To stretch, balance on the left foot, bringing the right foot up behind you toward your buttock, grab the forefoot with your hand, and stretch gently. Switch sides. Then stand on your left foot again and slide your right leg behind you, pressing the right leg toward the floor until you feel the stretch along the back of that leg. Switch sides.

LUNGES

This is a great exercise for toning the entire leg, but we do not recommend them if you have knee problems. There are a variety of versions, and with each version, you lunge by stepping with one leg and sinking down, which causes the knee of the stationary leg to bend. Switch sides to work both legs. Personal preference will determine if you prefer to alternate legs or do one set per leg and then change.

All of the lunges below start from a standing position; when you have done each one, return to a standing position.

- **Standing Lunge:** For this lunge, move your right leg straight back behind your body, flexing the right foot and sink down. This causes your left knee to bend. Switch legs.
- **Diagonal Lunge:** Move your right leg out at about a 45-degree angle and sink down. This again causes the left knee to bend.
- **Lateral Lunge:** Step the right knee out to the side and sink down, once again causing the left knee to bend. The important thing is to keep the left knee over the ankle.

CALF RAISES

This exercise will help create a more shapely lower leg. Stand with your feet slightly less than shoulder-width apart and hold on to a chair back or doorframe for balance. Rise up on your toes and come down again, stopping just short of your heels touching the floor. Repeat the motion with your heels together and toes pointing outward. To add challenge, you can alternate raising your heels and toes, or you can stand firmly on a stair in your home, letting your heel drop below the edge each time you come down. The most challenging version is to place one foot behind the ankle of your other leg, raise up, then come down, on one leg at a time.

 FAQS: FREQUENTLY ASKED QUESTIONS

AEROBIC EXERCISE - HOW MUCH IS ENOUGH?
Current research on interval aerobics, such as the Healthy Aging Interval Aerobics Workout recommended in this book, suggests that 25 minutes of regular interval aerobic training, conducted three days a week, will maintain a person's current level of aerobic fitness.

This is particularly important if you've lost fat on the Healthy Aging Program and want to keep it off. Low-intensity, long duration aerobics training will not necessarily burn more body fat

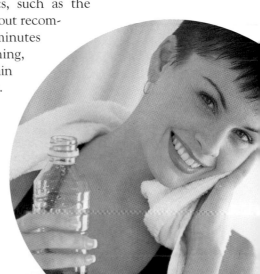

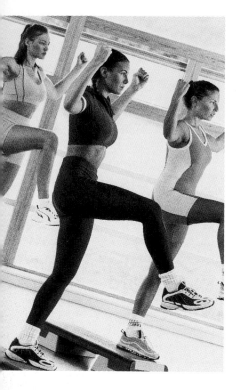

than high-intensity exercise. Remember, an interval aerobics program is not as concerned with how many calories you burn during the exercise as how many will be burned for up to an hour after the exercise. Remember also, when following this type of aerobics program, to conduct the exercise first thing in the morning on an empty stomach and try not to eat for one hour after the exercise.

A recent large-scale study, carried out by the Cooper Clinic and Institute for Aerobics Research in Dallas on 13,000 men and women over an eight-year time period, demonstrated that the least fit (those who lasted the shortest amount of time on the treadmill) had a far greater chance of dying prematurely from a chronic disease than those in all the other groups. The men in the highest fitness category had death rates that were about three-and-a half times lower than men in the low-fitness group.

The biggest improvement in the mortality-rate picture results from moving out of the lowest-fitness sedentary category into the next category, and it doesn't take much to make that transition. According to Dr. Steven Blair, lead researcher on the study, a 30 to 60 minute brisk daily walk will do it.

STRENGTH-CONDITIONING EXERCISE - HOW MUCH IS ENOUGH?

To maintain the muscle power you've gained, or already have, as indicated on your *Actual*Age™ results evaluation, you should conduct strength-training exercises three days per week, keeping the weight the same as in the last week of the program in Exercise Plan #3-Maintaining Fitness, and alternating upper and lower body workouts.

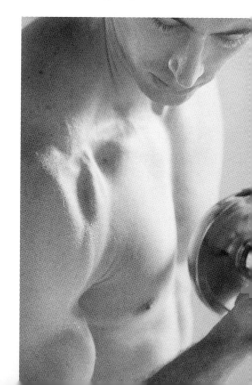

However, if you like the new toned and muscular contours of your body, you should push ahead and add to your muscle size and strength. To achieve that goal, you will need to continue to lift greater and greater weight, gradually.

At all times, your intensity should remain at about 80 percent of your maximal capacity, alternating upper and lower body workouts three days per week.

WHAT ARE THE SIGNS OF OVERTRAINING?

It is very important to start the *Actual*Age™ Exercise Plans slowly, and listen to your body as you begin to work out. You may be training too hard if you have some of the symptoms below:

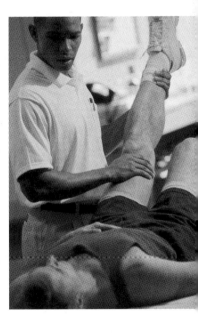

- Increased resting heart rate
- Frequent one-day colds
- Flu-like illnesses
- Increased incidence of infections
- Increased incidence of injuries
- Altered hormone status
- Loss of coordination
- Increased irritability and emotional sensitivity
- Sleep disturbances
- Decreased appetite
- Muscle soreness
- Decreased muscular strength
- Retarded return of blood pressure to basal levels after exercise
- Increased resting blood pressure

The best treatment for overtraining syndrome is prevention!

1. Allow 24 hours of recovery time between hard training sessions. For heavy weight training, you may need 48 hours or more for recovery, depending on your training level.

2. Get plenty of sleep (eight or more hours).

3. Eat a balanced diet.

4. If you cannot perform at the desired level or intensity that you had previously, either reduce intensity of training for that day or take a day off to rest.

5. Monitor your body signs and your resting heart rate.

6. Be aware of excessive muscle soreness and stiffness.

7. Be certain that you understand the importance of rest. Don't worry about taking a day or even a few days off to balance yourself.

IF I START WEIGHT LIFTING, WILL I LOOK LIKE A PROFESSIONAL WRESTLER?

No. There is no need to worry! About 99 percent of women and a significant percentage of men cannot develop huge muscles without spending hours and hours a day in the gym lifting serious weight. Most women don't have enough testosterone to add major bulk to their frames unless they take steroids.

Weight lifting may actually make you look smaller. Because muscle is a very compact, dense tissue, it takes up less room than fat. In the beginning, you may not lose any weight. You may even gain a few pounds, because muscle weighs more per square inch than fat. But you will notice that your clothes fit better. Don't look at your scale, look in your mirror for results.

IF I STOP LIFTING WEIGHTS, WON'T MY MUSCLE TURN TO FAT?

No. Fat and muscle are two very different substances. When you look at them under a microscope, fat looks like chicken coop wire and muscle looks like frayed electrical wiring. If you stop lifting weights, your muscles will simply shrink or atrophy.

HOW FAST SHOULD I DO MY REPS?

Reps or repetitions should take a full two seconds to lift a weight and two to four seconds to lower it. If you lift more quickly than that, you will end up relying on momentum rather than muscle power. Going slow and steady produces better results because more of your muscle gets "into the act."

HOW LONG SHOULD I REST BETWEEN SETS?

The amount of rest between sets can vary depending upon your training level. If you are a beginner, you should rest about 90 seconds between sets to give your muscles adequate time to recover. As you get in better shape, you need to rest less, between 30 to 60 seconds.

WHAT IF I GET SORE?

When you first begin the Healthy Aging Exercise Plans #2 and #3, which includes weight training, you can expect to feel a bit sore and tired afterward. (Keep in mind, if you have never done anything like this before, modest repetitions are the smart way to begin.) It is okay to "feel good about feeling sore!" Sore muscles are actually good because it means that your muscles are being used.

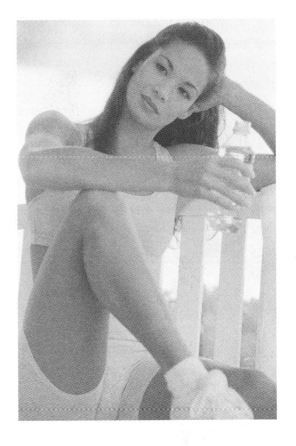

When you lift weights one day, we recommend you rest the following day. When you begin to strength train, you are actually creating small tears in the muscle fibers. This is what causes the soreness the day after you work out. The tears take two days to heal. This process results in a steady increase in your strength. The initial soreness will subside and be replaced by a feeling of post-exercise well-being. As you become more comfortable with strength training, you will begin to add more weight, and you may experience some soreness again. This is simply your muscles telling you that you have just gotten a bit stronger and a bit more fit than when you first began the program. A little bit of soreness is worth the small price you have to pay for the reward of the physical and emotional benefits you will receive.

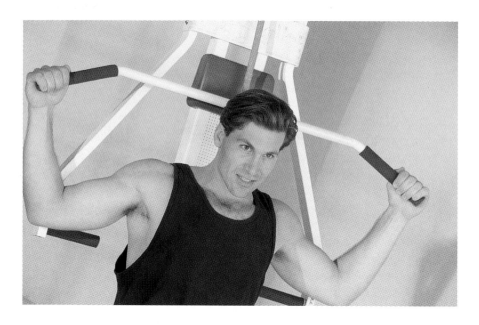

WHY SHOULD I CHALLENGE MYSELF?

With strength training, staying in your comfort zone won't allow you to become more fit very fast. If you just keep using an amount of weight that you can easily lift, you will maintain whatever muscle tone you have, but you won't steadily increase your strength. You have to challenge yourself. The **Actual**Age™ Healthy Aging Program recommends that you perform your strength-building exercises with weights or resistance that are about 80 percent of your one repetition maximum. Remember your one repetition maximum is the most weight you can lift with one try. In this way, you will be steadily increasing your weights as you increase your strength. At the same time, you will begin to experience how good you will feel when you work hard.

HOW DO MUSCLES HELP BURN FAT?

Strength training is the gift you give yourself that "keeps on giving!" With weight loss and fat reduction, your muscles keep working for you even after the workout is over. Exercising speeds up your metabolism. Researchers have found that a pound of muscle requires more calories than fat, even at rest. To you, this means that a fit and strong body uses more calories just to sustain itself than a person with more body fat, even when they weigh the same.

CONCLUSIONS

HEALTHY AGING REASSESSMENTS
Over the course of the 12 weeks, you'll be scheduled to retest your individual and overall **Actual**Age™ scores. Your healthcare provider will recommend the appropriate schedule for you to follow. By retaking the **Actual**Age™ evaluation at regular intervals and comparing the new results with the old, you'll be able to chart your progress far into the future.

WHAT IF YOU STOP THE HEALTHY AGING PROGRAM?
If you were forced to stop your Healthy Aging Program for any reason for longer than a month, you should go back and retake the **Actual**Age™ evaluation to find out what shape you're in. Your scores on the evaluation will place you into one of the Healthy Aging Exercise Plans. In that way, you will be able to restart your exercise program gradually. Following one of the Healthy Aging Exercise Plans is the safest way back to health and vitality.

THE EFFECTS OF EXERCISE ARE SHORT LIVED
Research by exercise physiologists indicate if you stop exercising, within one week many of the remarkable adaptations your muscles made due to exercise will be well on their way to being lost. The beneficial effects of exercise can't be stored. Exercise and body movement are intangible experiences that your body needs to undergo daily. Activity and good nutrition are the two fuels your body's engine must have in order to function normally. This is why the Healthy Aging Program is a program for life!

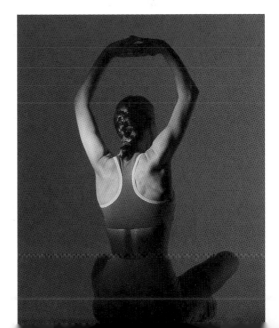

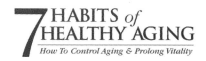

7 HABITS *of* HEALTHY AGING
How To Control Aging & Prolong Vitality

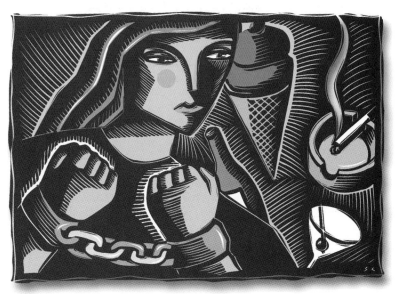

CHAPTER FOUR

Habit #4
Stimulants

KEY CONCEPT
Stimulants can become depressants which can lead to addiction. Regular use of stimulants can also raise your insulin levels and put you on a path for accelerated aging. Gradually reduce your use of stimulants, and the benefits can be more energy, increased concentration, more productivity, better sleep and an improved state of well-being.

Stimulant use has an indirect influence on excess insulin production and the eventual condition known as sarcopenia (age-related loss of muscle). By stimulant use, we are referring to the regular use of items like alcohol, caffeine, chocolate, sugar, excessive refined carbohydrates and tobacco.

Even though the goal of the Healthy Aging Program is to be off all stimulants, you must wean off stimulants gradually to avoid serious mood swings, depression and other withdrawal symptoms.

As you gradually reduce off stimulant use, if you find yourself irritable or depressed, increase your stimulant intake and continue to work on the other habits of Healthy Aging. As you become more balanced, slowly begin to decrease stimulant use again. Even though the goal is to be free of all stimulant use, you must recognize this process is a slow one that may require a lot of time.

Serotonin is one of the major neurotransmitter chemicals in the brain that affects mood and is responsible for communicating different needs between the brain and the body. Much like balancing insulin helps to balance other hormones in the body, balancing serotonin helps to balance the other neuro-transmitters.

When serotonin levels are normal, mood is good with a sense of well-being. Most people are energetic, productive, feel sharp, able to concentrate, sleep well, and wake refreshed.

When serotonin levels are at a steady low state, a person can experience anxiety, depression, loss of concentration and suffer from chronic insomnia.

This Healthy Aging Program which incorporates balanced eating and correct eating frequency, including proteins, fats and carbohydrates at each meal, will help provide ongoing serotonin production in the brain. Some of the serotonin is used immediately, and some is stored for future use. A diet high in carbohydrates and devoid of protein and fat will produce only a small amount of serotonin, resulting in too little to keep your moods balanced. Stress, caffeine, soft drinks, alcohol, tobacco and eating lots of sugar creates a low serotonin state, which ultimately increases the need for more stimulants, and marks the beginning of a vicious cycle.

HOW STIMULANTS ACCELERATE AGING

When you use stimulants or eat excessive carbohydrates, insulin levels rise. This results in a rapid release of serotonin from the storage supply in the brain, causing mood to significantly improve and a state of

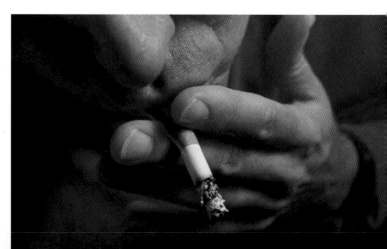

well-being to transpire. Even though this appears on the surface to be good, it's not. This "high" of stored serotonin is a temporary high that is quickly used up. When serotonin levels drop again, a person begins to feel down once more. This sets up a cycle of the symptoms of low serotonin and the need to eat an excess of carbohydrates or use more stimulants to once again obtain the high.

It becomes very easy to give in to the cravings created from low serotonin levels, which generally cannot be overcome by sheer willpower alone. People react differently to low serotonin levels. Whenever you are overcome with the urge to eat sweets, drink coffee or alcohol, or use tobacco, you now know that it is your brain responding to low serotonin levels.

HOW ALL STIMULANTS BECOME DEPRESSANTS

Caffeine use, for instance, causes the release of serotonin, which improves your mood. After a short while, your mood crashes from the drop in serotonin levels, and you experience additional cravings for more caffeine. This is the pattern regardless of the stimulant: caffeine, sugar, tobacco or alcohol, and this usually leads to an addiction.

Craving caffeine can cause craving for tobacco. Eating sugar can cause a craving for alcohol and so on. Anyone hooked on stimulants has been through this craving cycle. Basically, the use of any stimulant can make you dependent on other stimulants to get the high from the serotonin release. Eventually, a person will end up serotonin depleted and very depressed; this is why all stimulants eventually become depressants.

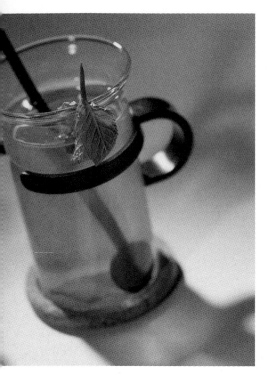

CAFFEINE

Most people are not aware of what happens if they drink tea, coffee or colas with caffeine in place of water. Caffeine in these products are central nervous system stimulants and, at the same time, dehydrating agents because of their strong diuretic action on the kidneys. One cup of coffee contains about 85 milligrams of caffeine, and one cup of tea or one cola drink contains about 50 milligrams. The effect of caffeine may at times be considered desirable, but constant substituting of caffeine-containing drinks for water will deprive the body of its full capacity for the formation of hydroelectric energy. Excess caffeine will also deplete the ATP-stored energy in the brain and the body, a possible contributing factor for shorter attention span in the younger, cola-consuming generation, or chronic fatigue syndrome as a result of excess coffee consumption in later life. Do not forget that dehydration is the number one stressor of the human body or any living matter.

COFFEE

Coffee is a narcotic beverage. The caffeine in coffee belongs to the same alkaloid group of chemicals as morphine, cocaine and strychnine. The caffeine combines with hydrochloric acid and forms a potent toxin, caffeine hydrochloride. As this toxin is absorbed into your portal circulation and hits your liver, bile is released in an attempt to flush it from your system. This is what accounts for the increase in bowel "regularity" of which many coffee drinkers boast. If you are one of these people, you might ask yourself, "Is such a toxin-induced flush really very health promoting?"

Drinking decaffeinated coffee is likely no better than drinking regular coffee because of the large concentration of the chemical trichloroethylene. It is a close relative of the plastic chemical vinyl chloride, which has been linked to certain types of liver cancer. Nitrosomines, which occur naturally in coffee beans, are the same co-carcinogens as those found in cured meats and bacon.

Heavy coffee drinkers create thiamine (B-1) insufficiency. Symptoms of B-1 insufficiency range from fatigue, nervousness, general malaise, general aches and pains to headaches. By the way, alcohol also depletes B-1 from your system.

Regular use of coffee is believed to destroy important vitamins and minerals. It also prevents some of the nutrients in your food from being absorbed effectively in your small intestine.

The "buzz" or stimulation one gets from coffee actually contributes to rebound fatigue when the stimulating effects wear off. Repeated stimulation can contribute to the exhaustion of key organs like the liver, pancreas and adrenal glands.

SOFT DRINKS

In 1994, the annual consumption of sodas per person in America, was 49.1 gallons. The vast numbers of people who drink sodas are drinking the caffeinated type. The soft drink association surveyed the use of soft drinks in hospitals in America and found 85 percent serve sodas with their patients' meals, even though research has shown that caffeine is addictive.

The broad-based increase in consumption of mainly caffeine-containing sodas forms the background to many of the health problems of our society. The mistaken assumption that all fluids are equivalent to water is the main cause of many of the ills of the human body. It is also frequently associated with the initial excessive gain in weight.

Caffeine, one of the main components of most sodas, coffee drinks and tea, is a drug. It has addictive properties because of its direct action on the brain. It also acts on the kidneys and causes increased urine production. Caffeine has diuretic properties and is physiologically a dehydrating agent. This characteristic is the main reason a person is forced to drink so many cans of soda every day and never be satisfied. The water does not stay in the body long enough. At the same time, many persons confuse their feeling of thirst for water as a hungry sensation. Thinking they have consumed enough "water" that is in the soda or coffee, they assume they are hungry and begin to eat more than their body's need for food. Thus, dehydration caused by caffeine-consumption, in due time, will cause a gradual gain in weight from overeating as a direct result over confusion of thirst and hunger sensations.

ALCOHOL

Alcohol doesn't contain any fat, but it is loaded with carbohydrates and empty calories. Just one gram of alcohol contains seven calories, nearly as much as a gram of fat. Consuming just two beers equates to about a fourth of the calories you should be taking for an entire day if your goal is to lose excess body fat. Most of the excess calories from alcohol are not needed by your body for energy and are thus promptly stored as fat. Several studies have shown drinking alcohol socially contributes to abdominal fat accumulation. A Swedish study that compared recreational drinkers with nondrinkers found that the recreational drinkers had two to three times the amount of abdominal fat.

HOW TO STOP STIMULANT CRAVINGS NATURALLY

In order to put an end to these type of cravings and help with moody conditions, you must make sure your body has everything the brain needs to produce serotonin on an ongoing basis. To provide the essentials you need, you must follow the Balanced Eating Habit #1 that supplies enough good protein, fat and carbohydrates to balance insulin and the other hormones of the body. You must also make sure you receive enough B vitamins, calcium and magnesium from your diet or from supplementation. Both vitamin B and magnesium are used up in the body when stimulants are used regularly. You must also stop the habits that reduce serotonin. When the brain is able to produce enough serotonin on a continuous basis to keep a positive mood level, your brain will stop demanding items that will stimulate quick serotonin releases from its storage sites.

INCREASE CONSUMPTION OF PURE WATER

Ensure that you consume approximately two liters or eight cups of pure water each day. Consider drinking the majority of your water between meals in order to prevent any interference with digestion. Since the water we drink provides for cell function and its volume requirements, the decrease in our daily water intake affects the efficiency of cell activity. It is the reason for the loss of water volume held inside the cells of the body.

HEALTHY AGING

Excess carbohydrates and stimulants used to alleviate the symptoms of low serotonin contribute to chronic high insulin levels. Stress also causes the release of insulin. It's important to correct all behaviors that cause low serotonin in order to keep insulin levels balanced and to maintain a positive mood level.

Low serotonin levels can be balanced. When you realize that one imbalance in the body leads to another imbalance, you suddenly realize that the 7 Habits outlined in this book are key to Healthy Aging and your well-being. If you follow balanced eating, eating frequency and begin to reduce stimulants, your body can begin to correct your low serotonin levels. Eventually, you will find that you no longer crave carbohydrates and no longer suffer from depression, poor concentration and the lack of excitement in life. The only way to recover from excess stimulant use and a low serotonin state is to get started and through the process, and remember that it does take time.

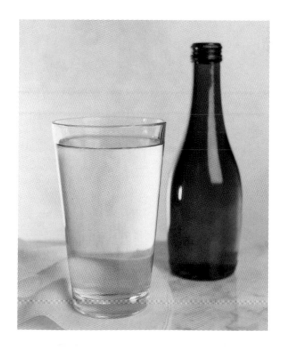

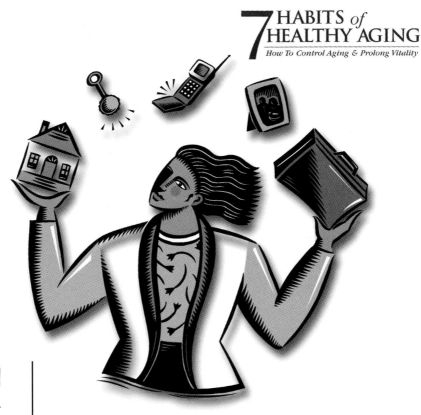

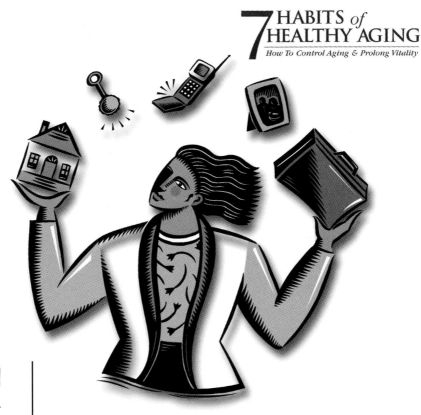

7 HABITS *of*
HEALTHY AGING
How To Control Aging & Prolong Vitality

CHAPTER FIVE

Habit #5
Stress

KEY CONCEPT
Mental/emotional stress imbalances every hormone system in your body and contributes to ill health. Stress weakens your resistance, increases the chance of disease, contributes to fat gain and puts you on the fast track to aging. Proper rest and stress reduction will help you increase your health and vitality.

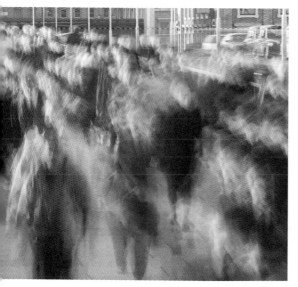

Stress has an indirect influence on excess insulin production and the eventual condition known as sarcopenia (age-related loss of muscle), through the stimulation of hormones know as adrenaline and cortisol.

Stress is harmful because stress imbalances every hormone system of your body. The imbalances are apparent in the way you feel during periods of stress or right after a stressful situation. To achieve Healthy Aging, you must focus on regular stress management to keep insulin and other hormone levels balanced.

Stress on a daily basis can feel like too much to deal with. There are, however, many ways to get relief through the use of stress management that can help provide a greater sense of balance.

Times of stress require extreme discipline to keep the other Healthy Aging Habits like balanced eating, eating frequency and stimulant use under control. If you find yourself in a stressful situation, stop momentarily and look to see what you can do to maintain your current level of health.

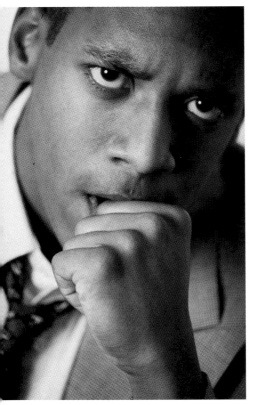

SEROTONIN LEVELS AND STRESS

Another important factor that leads to low serotonin states is mental/emotional stress. Mental/emotional stress depletes serotonin levels without the initial "high" release that you get from using other stimulants. During times of emotional stress, it is important to make sure that you eat well and take extra care to replenish your serotonin levels by following Habits #1, #2 and #3. If you do not, it can lead to depression and cravings for other stimulants.

STRESS ADDICTION

Mental/emotional stress is not the same as stress you put yourself into in pressure situations. Some people are "addicted" to stress and pressure because they love the release of stress hormones like adrenaline, insulin and cortisol, which stimulate the brain to release serotonin. With the release of serotonin, they suddenly focus better, think more quickly, and become more productive. When the stress is over, serotonin levels drop and so does the high feeling. These types of people continue to look for pressure situations to experience the high all over again. Being addicted to stress is also very unhealthy. Stress management is vital to maintaining balanced serotonin levels. Since it takes time to regenerate serotonin, it is important to give your brain a rest from stress. This is best accomplished through proper rest periods, adequate sleep and good stress management techniques.

Stress is a part of life. It is up to you to do whatever is necessary to manage your particular problem in the best way to suit your needs. If stress is a major factor in your life, you must seek out professional counseling. At the end of this section are some simple, yet effective, ways to reduce stress from everyday situations. Be sure to add any of the activities to your daily schedule that you feel are appropriate for you.

In order to maximize your benefit from participating in the Healthy Aging Program, you need to be aware of the various factors that add to your stress load, weaken your resistance and can lead to fat gain, muscle loss and disease.

Health can best be understood as a state of balance. The more balanced and centered you are, the more readily and appropriately you can respond to the various stressors and demands which you face day in and day out. In order to regain and maintain a more balanced and healthful state, you must be able to recognize those factors in your lifestyle that stress you and get you out of balance.

THE FOUR VECTORS OF STRESS

There are four key areas or vectors of stress to be considered: mental/emotional, nutritional/chemical, physical/structural and electromagnetic. With a more

comprehensive understanding of the four vectors of stress, you will be able to begin differentiating the contributing factors to any condition you experience at any given time. Through the more skillful recognition of the contributing factors or causes of an ailment, you will have taken the first crucial step in its resolution.

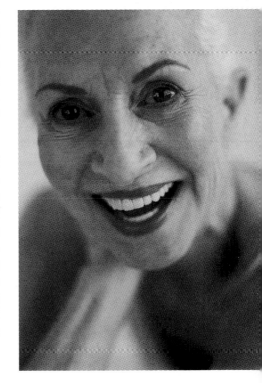

Although proficiency in the area of "stress awareness" may take some practice to accomplish, your efforts will be uniquely rewarding. Clear patterns of the stressors that are precipitating your health challenges will become apparent. This will provide the clear direction you require, allowing you to focus on the development of the lifestyle skills required to resolve your key stressors and to strengthen your specific resistance to them.

STRESS-INDUCED INSOMNIA

Insomnia is a major problem in society. The epidemic of insomnia stems from a low serotonin state. Serotonin is converted to melatonin in the pineal gland in the brain. Melatonin is one of the important hormones that help you get to sleep and stay asleep all night. Any of the factors that contribute to a low-serotonin state can contribute to a low-melatonin state. You need a balanced eating program that includes protein, fats and carbohydrates at every meal to make hormones such as cortisol, estrogen, and testosterone, to help regulate melatonin production. If you do not eat enough food by utilizing a proper-eating frequency, you will also contribute to insomnia by decreasing serotonin production and increasing adrenaline levels.

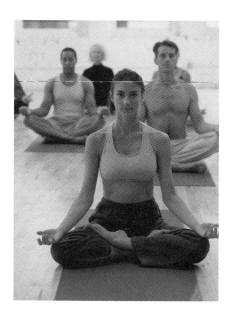

PROPER REST DURING THE DAY TO REDUCE STRESS

Proper rest is the freedom from disturbance of mind or spirit and the presence of peace of mind. How then may we better cope with stress? While most of us are aware of the need for a good night's sleep, too few recognize the need for proper rest during the day. Both those who are engaged in heavy physical labor and business executives or white collar workers alike are subjected to a variety of physical stressors throughout their working hours. There is mounting evidence that those who manage to obtain proper rest and more resourceful postures during the day not only live more comfortably and work more effectively, they also live longer. Once convinced of the benefit, how does one go about obtaining proper rest during the business hours? Proper rest refers to those inactivities that serve to aid restoration of optimal mental and physical function, in other words, good health. Your goal here is to assist your nervous system in its ability to cope with the variety of stresses imposed upon it, and assist the physical body in compensating for the wear and tear of manual activities and the effects of gravity. All that is normally required is 15 to 20 minutes, twice daily, in addition to your usual night's sleep, to counteract the onslaught of stress-related fatigue and wear and tear. There are various books and classes in nearly every community on learning how to meditate, a very beneficial way of acquiring proper body rest during the day.

SIMPLE WAYS TO REDUCE STRESS

- Join a stress management class.

- Learn to meditate.

- Learn to practice yoga.

- Get plenty of sleep.

- Avoid stressful movies
  and television programs.

- Balance work and relaxation time.

- Have dinner with your
  family on a regular basis.

- Learn how to say "no".

- Join a health club.

- Develop affection in relationships.

- Laugh more and hug more.

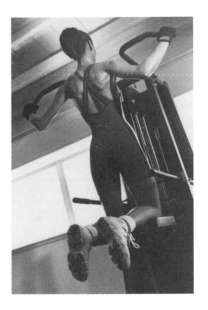

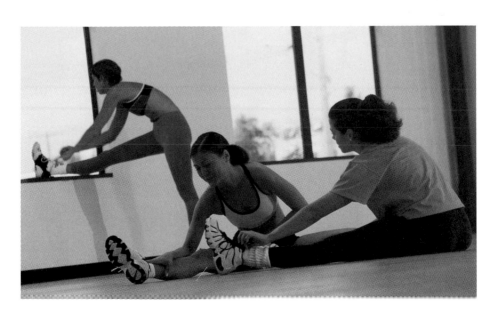

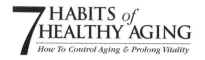
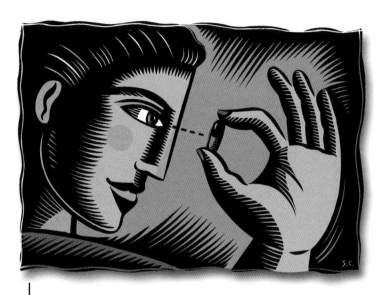

CHAPTER SIX

Habit #6
Supplements

KEY CONCEPT

With today's fast-paced, fast-food lifestyle, proper supplementation can be one of the most dynamic opportunities to improve your health. High quality supplements can help you achieve and maintain proper body composition, help slow the aging process and help ensure improved health and vitality.

Supplements can be extremely valuable aids to Healthy Aging. It's almost impossible to get all the nutrients your body needs to remain healthy, support recovery from exercise and stress, and increase muscle mass from food alone. Supplements are often more convenient than whole foods, and high quality, ratio-balanced meal replacements allow you to get in those extra meals every day.

Supplemental meal replacements let you control your protein, carbohydrate and fat intake conveniently, and they're especially valuable in enabling you to greatly increase protein intake without a commensurate rise in fat intake.

Periods of high stress from work or exercise can create a need for the various benefits that can be derived from substances not normally found in food or produced in the body in sufficient quantities.

A high quality multivitamin-mineral, additional antioxidants, joint-support supplements that contain glucosamine and chondroitin, essential fatty acids and body composition products should be standard issue for anyone who hopes to benefit the most from the Healthy Aging Program.

WHAT DOES A (BIA) BODY COMPOSITION DETECT?

Historically the most accurate methods of determining body composition have either been inaccurate, cumbersome or too expensive. Fortunately, a technique called Bioelectrical Impedance Analysis (BIA) makes the accurate assessment of body composition available to everyone. It's simple, fast, inexpensive and accurate. In fact, independent researchers have found bioimpedance to be a highly reliable method of assessing body composition with a retest accuracy of 99 percent.

Bioelectrical Impedance Analysis (BIA) identifies changes in body composition at such an early stage that it can be treated effectively and efficiently. It is a proactive measurement, rather than a reactive one. The electrical properties of a system like the body make it possible to assess total body fat, muscle mass, body water and its associated intercellular and extracellular compartments.

The applications for this kind of evaluation by healthcare providers are many. BIA body compositions can be used as part of a routine physical exam or to monitor changes in muscle mass in the Healthy Aging Program.

SUPPLEMENT USE AND (BIA) BODY COMPOSITION

The area of nutritional medicine and supplementation represents perhaps one of the most dynamic opportunities for health improvement today, and proper body composition is vital to good health. Body composition and the volume of fluids and tissues change with a person's nutritional state. Maintaining a healthy body composition, not weight, is a key ingredient to optimal health. The proper lean body mass-to-body fat ratios have been associated with longevity and reduced risks for cardiovascular disease and cancer. Achieving a natural balance maintains health, improves recovery and enhances your overall well-being.

CORRECT SUPPLEMENTATION CAN LEAD TO IMPROVED BODY COMPOSITION

If you're the average, middle-aged person, your problem is not excess weight so much as it is excess body fat coupled with too little muscle. If you want to avoid the decreasing muscle/increasing fat disease state called sarcopenia (age-related loss of muscle), it's imperative that you look beyond the simplistic notion of losing weight.

The 7 Healthy Aging Habits listed in this book are asking you to focus not on body fat versus muscle, but instead concentrate on building muscle at the expense of fat. The crux of the matter is a concept called body composition and the necessary lifestyle changes and supplements needed to effect a positive change.

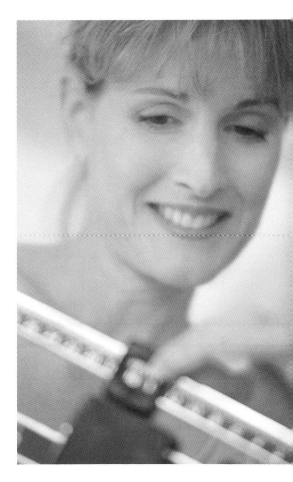

WHAT DOES A BIA BODY COMPOSITION SHOW?

Scientists divide the components of the body into two broad categories, body fat and lean body mass. The former is just what the term implies, fat, known also as adipose tissue. The latter is everything that is not fat: bone and other vital organ tissues, your central nervous system and so on. It mostly consists of muscle.

Body fat is metabolically inactive; it is energy-storage tissue. It's been implicated in a broad range of chronic and potentially lethal diseases including diabetes, hypertension, heart disease and now, sarcopenia. Muscle, bone and vital organs (lean-body mass) are the body's biologically active tissue. This tissue, especially muscle,

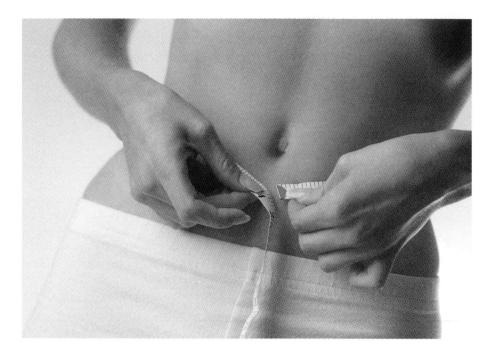

needs a far greater amount of caloric fuel to maintain itself compared to body fat. People with a high ratio of muscle-to-fat have a higher metabolism and a higher calorie need. On the other hand, fewer calories are needed to maintain fat tissue, so obese people have a lower metabolism and a harder time losing weight no matter how little they eat. In addition, people who are accumulating fat are simultaneously lowering muscular strength because the muscle component of lean-body mass is lost at a more rapid rate than any of the other components.

Muscle, to a far greater extent than most people realize, is responsible for the vitality of your whole physiological apparatus. It's why muscle mass and strength are considered the top two biomarkers of aging and why building muscle is the key to rejuvenation.

A strong, toned musculature makes all sorts of wonderful contributions to your overall well-being. A high ratio of muscle-to-fat on the body causes the metabolism to rise, meaning you can more easily burn body fat and alter your body composition even further in favor of beneficial muscle tissue. It triggers muscle to use more insulin, thus greatly reducing the chances you'll ever develop diabetes, and it helps maintain higher levels of the beneficial HDL cholesterol in your blood.

BIOMARKERS OF AGING
Three of the top biomarkers of aging, muscle mass, basal metabolic rate and body fat, which are the primary catalysts for preventing sarcopenia (age-related loss of muscle), can be measured and monitored by getting a body composition analysis using bioelectrical impedance (BIA).

SPECIFIC SUPPLEMENTS USING (BIA) BODY COMPOSITION AS A GUIDE
Specific supplements can better be recommended after a thorough body composition is conducted, especially if the evaluation is able to identify the key biomarkers of aging. Additionally, body composition results are best used for tracking long-term nutritional trends. A series of BIA tests over several months can provide a trend that will show whether your health is improving, declining or staying the same, which enables you to adjust your supplement program accordingly.

The Healthy Aging Program outlined in this book will put you on the path to optimal health and ideal body composition through a combination of balanced eating, eating frequency, reduction of stimulants and stress, and using the correct supplements to control aging and prolong vitality.

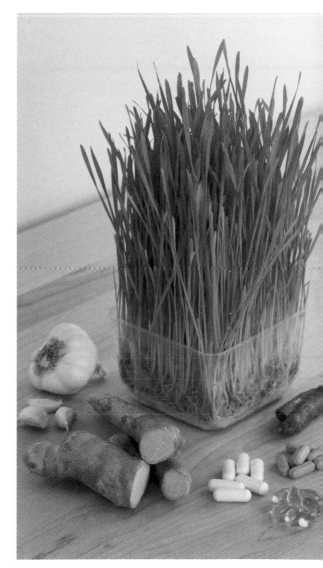

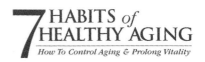

7 HABITS *of* HEALTHY AGING
How To Control Aging & Prolong Vitality

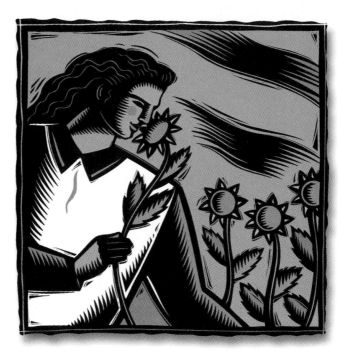

CHAPTER SEVEN

Habit #7
Hormone Balance

KEY CONCEPT

Hormones in your body work in harmony. Just as it is not healthy to have high or low thyroid levels, it is not healthy to have high or low insulin levels. To maintain optimal health, all hormones should be in balance. The best way to achieve hormone balance is to first adhere to the first six habits in this program. If further hormone optimization is needed, consult your physician or healthcare provider for guidance.

THE 7 HABITS OF HEALTHY AGING

This program is designed to help men and women balance their health habits and improve every aspect of their lives. The best way to achieve this goal is through incorporating the first six habits of this program.

If, after following a balanced eating program, improving your eating frequency, adopting an exercise plan, eliminating stimulants, managing your stress and optimizing your nutritional supplement intake, you still do not reach maximum vitality and the ideal body composition, you may have a hormone imbalance. This is because the loss of hormones is part of the normal aging process.

NATURAL HORMONE OPTIMIZATION

If implementing the first six habits of this book has not achieved the vitality and vigor expected, perhaps you can achieve your goal through the added synergy of hormone optimization with human growth stimulation by using natural oral secretagogues, along with the other six habits.

Your healthcare provider is best suited to decide how to proceed with hormone optimization. Be sure to schedule an appointment and discuss your options. Never attempt hormone optimization or hormone replacement therapy without first consulting your physician or healthcare provider.

HORMONE REPLACEMENT THERAPY

If the decision has been made to proceed with hormone replacement therapy, be sure to seek out a physician who is well versed in hormone replacement therapy and who uses real hormones that are identical to the hormones found in the human body.

The systems of the human body are all linked together and work synergistically. When there is one imbalance, it creates another imbalance, which leads to stress, degeneration, and eventually premature aging. All the systems of the body should be balanced, including all of your hormones.

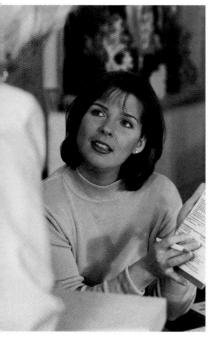

HEALTH TAKES TIME – BUT IT'S WORTH IT

It takes time to change habits of accelerated aging and turn them around to healthy ones; you cannot achieve metabolic balance overnight.

If you think how many years it has taken to get to your current state, you should be able to understand why it must take time to repair. The good news is, it usually requires much less time to repair than it took to breakdown, provided you follow the Healthy Aging Habits. Be patient. For most people, the hardest part is changing the lifestyle habits necessary to receive the health benefits they desire. Do not get frustrated or discouraged. It can take 12 to 18 months or more to slow down and reverse the damage caused by years of accelerated aging abuse. If you stick to the program, you will, at some time, agree the effort was worth it.

As you follow the 7 Habits of Healthy Aging: balanced eating, eating frequency, exercise, removal of stimulants, reduction of stress, optimization of supplements, and finally reach hormone balance, you will realize how wonderful it is to be able to control your aging and prolong your vitality.

You will benefit in many ways: more energy, better sleep, less body fat, more strength, reduced cravings for stimulants, healthier skin, nails and hair, fewer aches and pains, and a renewed vigor and vitality.

This may be the end of the book, but it is just the beginning for you! I hope you continue your journey to better health long after these words have been read.

Good luck. Health and vitality are your birthright. Access it and live your life to the fullest!

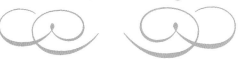

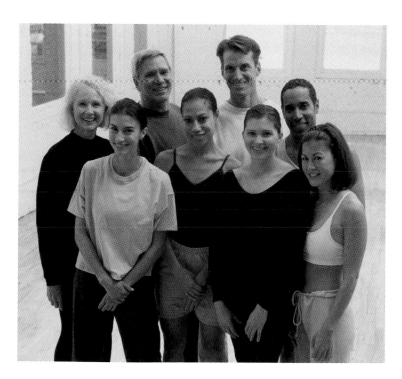

THE *ACTUAL*AGE™ ASSESSMENT

Keep in mind that chronology is not destiny. Your body is not necessarily aging on the same timetable as that of your peers. Indeed, different organ systems within your own body may be aging at widely divergent rates. This distinction between your body's chronological age and its biological age is a very important one. The **Actual**Age™ Assessment may prove to be one of the most important evaluations you make for yourself and your entire family.

WHAT IS THE *ACTUAL*AGE™ ASSESSMENT?

ActualAge™ is a patent pending, breakthrough assessment procedure that helps measure and track healthy aging. Using internationally recognized tests, a state-of-the-art diagnostic evaluation called a bioimpedance analysis, and scientifically derived algorithms, **Actual**Age™ assesses five major areas of healthy aging: lean body mass, body strength, body shape, body fat and the heart. These five isolated age scores are then combined to calculate an overall **Actual**Age™.

The objective in the **Actual**Age™ Assessment is to compare your chronological age with the biological age of your body.

Ultimately, your **Actual**Age™ should equal or be younger than your chronological age. For example, an active 40-year-old may have an **Actual**Age™ of 30 (comparable to the health and fitness of a 30-year-old); an inactive 40-year-old may have an **Actual**Age™ of 50.

WHY DISCOVER YOUR *ACTUAL*AGE™?

Your chronological age is fixed, but your **Actual**Age™ may be older or younger depending on a combination of factors. **Actual**Age™ results help you understand where you're doing well and where you can improve, in order to increase vitality and promote healthy aging. You'll discover that knowing your age in "healthy aging" years is a unique motivational force that provides a tangible incentive to establish and maintain positive health habits.

Regular **Actual**Age™ testing will help track and monitor your progress over time, which can provide added motivation for anyone trying to:
• Slow Down Accelerated Aging
• Lose Weight
• Improve Body Shape
• Reduce Stress
• Increase Energy

After receiving an **Actual**Age™ Assessment you'll receive your results in a manner that is easy to understand and informative. This will provide an immediate motivational boost to either maintain or improve your current state of health and vitality.

WHAT IS USED TO MEASURE MY *ACTUAL*AGE™?

Research on aging at a major university in Boston listed several key "biomarkers of aging" in order of importance that can be measured, monitored and improved through lifestyle changes. The diagnostic equipment in the **Actual**Age™ Program used to assess your body's age measures several of these key biomarkers. The **Actual**Age™ evaluation itself is non-invasive, painless and takes only a few minutes.

HOW DOES MY *ACTUAL*AGE™ SCORE
DETERMINE THE BEST EXERCISE PLAN FOR ME?

Once your overall **Actual**Age™ score is established, one of the following three exercise plans should be implemented.

• EXERCISE PLAN #1: LOW FIT – (16 WEEK PLAN)
Your overall **Actual**Age™ score is 10 years or more above your chronological age. Four weeks aerobics only program for the low fit. Then move to Exercise Plan #2. Follow the instructions for this plan in Chapter 3.

• EXERCISE PLAN #2: MODERATELY FIT – (12 WEEK PLAN)
Your overall **Actual**Age™ score is one to nine years above your chronological age. This Exercise Plan is a 12-week, midcourse correction plan consisting of aerobic, strength and flexibility exercises for the moderately fit. Follow the instructions for this plan which are located in Chapter 3, then move to Exercise Plan #3.

• EXERCISE PLAN #3: MAINTAINING FITNESS (PLAN FOR LIFE)
Your overall **Actual**Age™ score is equal to your chronological age or below. You either measured this way initially or successfully reduced your **Actual**Age™ score by following Exercise Plan #1 (16-week plan) or Exercise Plan #2 (12-week plan). Either way, Exercise Plan #3 is a lifelong program that includes aerobic, strength and flexibility exercises to maintain your fitness level. Follow the instructions for this plan located in Chapter 3.

THE GOAL OF THE HEALTHY AGING PROGRAM IS HORMONE BALANCE: WHEN ALL OF THE HABITS ARE PRACTICED IN HARMONY, HORMONE BALANCE AND, ULTIMATELY, BETTER HEALTH WILL BE ACHIEVED.

***ACTUAL*AGE™ CASE STUDY**

Following is an example of a 51-year-old male, with no initial complaints who had his ***Actual*Age™** Assessment conducted.

On February, 3, 2001, the patient's ***Actual*Age™** was evaluated at 31 years old, as compared to his chronological age of 51. Since his ***Actual*Age™** was 20 years lower than his real age, he was advised to follow the 7 Habits of Healthy Aging guidelines and use Exercise Plan #3.

After 16 weeks on the Healthy Aging Program, the patient had his ***Actual*Age™** Assessment redone and found the following changes.

He gained 3.6 pounds of valuable muscle, while at the same time losing 1.6 pounds of body fat. His basal metabolic rate increased from 1841 calories to 1894 calories, which indicates that he will now burn more fat at rest. His total body water increased by 2 liters, because muscle is mostly water. Since the patient gained nearly 4 pounds of muscle, he would be expected to have higher total body water. The patient's weight went up 2 pounds, because muscle weighs more than fat; at the same time, he improved his body shape, as determined by a reduction in his waist-to-hip ratio measurement.

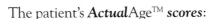

The patient's ***Actual*Age™ *scores*:**

- Muscle age improved by 3 years
- Strength age improved by 17 years
- Body fat age improved by 3 years
- Body shape age improved by 9 years
- Heart age improved by 15 years

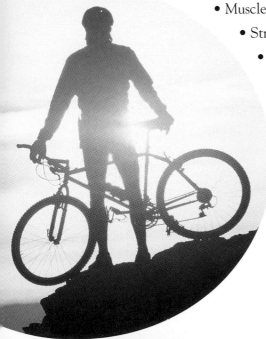

Results of the case study:
In only four months, the patient was able to reduce his ***Actual*Age™** score from 31 to 21 years, or in essence, "buy back" 10 years of health and vitality!

*Actual*Age™ CASE STUDY

Client Age:	51
Main Complaint:	None
Initial **Actual**Age™:	31 2-3-01
Ending **Actual**Age™:	21 5-19-01
Length of Program:	16 weeks
Program Followed:	Healthy Aging Program Plan #3

BIA RESULTS	BEFORE	AFTER	CHANGES
Muscle Mass:	130.1 lbs. 83.5%	133.7 lbs. 84.7%	+3.6 lbs.
Body Fat:	25.9 lbs. 16.5%	24.3 lbs. 15.3%	-1.6 lbs.
Basal Metabolic Rate:	1841 cals	1894 cals	+53 cals
Total Body Water:	42.5 liters	44.5 liters	+2.0 liters
Intracellular Water:	23.5 liters 53.3%	25.8 liters 58.0%	+2.3 liters
Body Weight:	156 lbs.	158 lbs.	+2.0 lbs.

ActualAge™ RESULTS	BEFORE	AFTER	CHANGES
Muscle Age	24 years	21 years	3 years younger
Strength Age	35 years	18 years	17 years younger
Body Fat Age	24 years	21 years	3 years younger
Body Shape Age	33 years	24 years	9 years younger
Heart Age	37 years	22 years	15 years younger
ActualAge™ Total	31 Years	21 Years	10 Years Younger

FIGURE 3

PERSONAL PROGRAM RECOMMENDATIONS

Name:_____ Date:_____

Provided By:_____ Phone:_____

Please review and adhere to the following recommendations:

❏ **Habit #1 Balanced Eating**
A balanced meal is a meal that has all three of the major macronutrients present: carbohydrates, fats and protein. Each meal should consist of 15 grams of protein, 20 grams of complex carbohydrates and 6-7 grams of healthy oils. Review the information and instructions in Chapter 1.

❏ **Habit #2 Eating Frequency**
Following is your daily protein requirement. Divide your meals evenly throughout the day, consuming approximately 15 grams of protein with each meal, whether it is real food, a meal-replacement shake or a nutrition bar.

> Daily Protein Requirement: _____ grams per day
> Daily Eating Frequency: _____ meals per day

> If the number of meals required per day proves to be too many for your lifestyle, then you may double up at one or more meals by consuming up to 30 grams of protein, 40 grams of complex carbohydrates, and 12-14 grams of healthy oils per meal. Never eat less than 5 meals that contain 15 grams of protein each, in order to maintain a minimum of 800 calories per day.

> **Balanced Meal Replacements (MR)**

> ❏ 1 MR Shake/Day   ❏ 2 MR Shakes/Day   ❏ 3 MR Shakes/Day   ❏ 4 MR Shakes/Day

> Other:_____
> Review the information and instructions in Chapter 2.

❏ **Habit #3 Regular Exercise**
Regular exercise along with proper diet will increase your vitality and slow down the aging process.

> ❏ **Exercise Plan #1- Low Fit (16-Week Plan)**

> *Actual*Age™ score is 10 years or more above your chronological age. Four-week aerobics only program for the low fit. Then move to Plan #2. Follow the instructions for this plan in Chapter 3.

> ❏ **Exercise Plan #2- Moderately Fit (12-Week Plan)**

> *Actual*Age™ score is one to nine years or more above your chronological age. Twelve-week aerobic, strength and flexibility program for the moderately fit. Then move to Plan #3. Follow the instructions for this plan in Chapter 3.

❏ **Exercise Plan #3- Maintaining Fitness (Plan for Life!)**
*Actual*Age™ score equals your chronological age or below. You either measured this way initially or successfully reduced your *Actual*Age™ score by following the 12 or 16-week plans. Either way, Plan #3 is a nutritionally sound, lifestyle-enhanced program that includes aerobic, strength and flexibility maintenance programs to use for life to prevent returning to a low or moderately fit condition. Follow the instructions for this plan in Chapter 3.

❏ **Your Heart Rate Zone (Found in Chapter 3)**
220 Minus Your Age=Your Maximum Heart Rate (MHR)

220 minus _____(age) = _____ (MHR)
❏ Exercise Plan # 1 = MHR multiplied by .50 percent
_____ (MHR) X 0.5 = _____ Beats per Minute (BPM)

❏ Exercise Plan # 2 = MHR multiplied by .60 percent
_____ (MHR) X 0.6 = _____ Beats per Minute (BPM)

❏ Exercise Plan # 3 = MHR multiplied by .70 percent
_____ (MHR) X 0.7 = _____ Beats per Minute (BPM)

❏ **Habit #4 Stimulants -** Gradually reduce your use of stimulants. The benefits can be more energy, increased concentration, more productivity, better sleep and an improved state of well-being. Review the information and instructions in Chapter 4.

Gradually reduce the following stimulants: ❏ Tobacco ❏ Alcohol ❏ Coffee
❏ Tea ❏ Soda ❏ Other_____

❏ **Habit #5 Stress Management -** For optimum health, regular stress management keeps insulin and other hormones balanced. Review the information and instructions in Chapter 5. Consider implementing one or more of the following:
❏ 20-minute walk in nature ❏ Outside deep breathing ❏ Feet up rest breaks ❏ Meditation
❏ Relaxing music break
❏ Other_____

❏ **Habit #6 Supplements -** High quality supplements can help you achieve and maintain proper body composition, slow the aging process and ensure improved health and vitality.

❏ Adhere to supplement recommendations listed on your Personalized Nutrition Prescription

❏ Other/Notes:_____
_____

❏ **Habit #7 Hormone Balance -** This is the ultimate goal of the Healthy Aging Program: when all the Habits are practiced in harmony, enormous health benefits will result. You will feel better, look better and add years to your life and life to your years!

Notes:_____
_____

PERSONAL PROGRAM RECOMMENDATIONS

Name:_____ Date:_____

Provided By:_____ Phone:_____

Please review and adhere to the following recommendations:

❏ **Habit #1 Balanced Eating**
A balanced meal is a meal that has all three of the major macronutrients present: carbohydrates, fats and protein. Each meal should consist of 15 grams of protein, 20 grams of complex carbohydrates and 6-7 grams of healthy oils. Review the information and instructions in Chapter 1.

❏ **Habit #2 Eating Frequency**
Following is your daily protein requirement. Divide your meals evenly throughout the day, consuming approximately 15 grams of protein with each meal, whether it is real food, a meal-replacement shake or a nutrition bar.

Daily Protein Requirement: _____ grams per day
Daily Eating Frequency: _____ meals per day

If the number of meals required per day proves to be too many for your lifestyle, then you may double up at one or more meals by consuming up to 30 grams of protein, 40 grams of complex carbohydrates, and 12-14 grams of healthy oils per meal. Never eat less than 5 meals that contain 15 grams of protein each, in order to maintain a minimum of 800 calories per day.

Balanced Meal Replacements (MR)

❏ 1 MR Shake/Day ❏ 2 MR Shakes/Day ❏ 3 MR Shakes/Day ❏ 4 MR Shakes/Day

Other:_____
Review the information and instructions in Chapter 2.

❏ **Habit #3 Regular Exercise**
Regular exercise along with proper diet will increase your vitality and slow down the aging process.

❏ **Exercise Plan #1- Low Fit (16-Week Plan)**
*Actual*Age™ score is 10 years or more above your chronological age. Four-week aerobics only program for the low fit. Then move to Plan #2. Follow the instructions for this plan in Chapter 3.

❏ **Exercise Plan #2- Moderately Fit (12-Week Plan)**
*Actual*Age™ score is one to nine years or more above your chronological age. Twelve-week aerobic, strength and flexibility program for the moderately fit. Then move to Plan #3. Follow the instructions for this plan in Chapter 3.

❏ **Exercise Plan #3- Maintaining Fitness (Plan for Life!)**

*Actual*Age™ score equals your chronological age or below. You either measured this way initially or successfully reduced your *Actual*Age™ score by following the 12 or 16-week plans. Either way, Plan #3 is a nutritionally sound, lifestyle-enhanced program that includes aerobic, strength and flexibility maintenance programs to use for life to prevent returning to a low or moderately fit condition. Follow the instructions for this plan in Chapter 3.

❏ **Your Heart Rate Zone (Found in Chapter 3)**

220 Minus Your Age=Your Maximum Heart Rate (MHR)

220 minus _____(age) = _____ (MHR)
❏ Exercise Plan # 1 = MHR multiplied by .50 percent
_____ (MHR) X 0.5 = _____ Beats per Minute (BPM)

❏ Exercise Plan # 2 = MHR multiplied by .60 percent
_____ (MHR) X 0.6 = _____ Beats per Minute (BPM)

❏ Exercise Plan # 3 = MHR multiplied by .70 percent
_____ (MHR) X 0.7 = _____ Beats per Minute (BPM)

❏ **Habit #4 Stimulants -** Gradually reduce your use of stimulants. The benefits can be more energy, increased concentration, more productivity, better sleep and an improved state of well-being. Review the information and instructions in Chapter 4.

Gradually reduce the following stimulants: ❏ Tobacco ❏ Alcohol ❏ Coffee
❏ Tea ❏ Soda ❏ Other_____

❏ **Habit #5 Stress Management -** For optimum health, regular stress management keeps insulin and other hormones balanced. Review the information and instructions in Chapter 5. Consider implementing one or more of the following:
❏ 20-minute walk in nature ❏ Outside deep breathing ❏ Feet up rest breaks ❏ Meditation
❏ Relaxing music break
❏ Other_____

❏ **Habit #6 Supplements -** High quality supplements can help you achieve and maintain proper body composition, slow the aging process and ensure improved health and vitality.

❏ Adhere to supplement recommendations listed on your Personalized Nutrition Prescription

❏ Other/Notes:_____
_____

❏ **Habit #7 Hormone Balance -** This is the ultimate goal of the Healthy Aging Program: when all the Habits are practiced in harmony, enormous health benefits will result. You will feel better, look better and add years to your life and life to your years!

Notes:_____
_____

PERSONAL PROGRAM RECOMMENDATIONS

Name:_____ Date:_____

Provided By:_____ Phone:_____

Please review and adhere to the following recommendations:

❏ **Habit #1 Balanced Eating**
A balanced meal is a meal that has all three of the major macronutrients present: carbohydrates, fats and protein. Each meal should consist of 15 grams of protein, 20 grams of complex carbohydrates and 6-7 grams of healthy oils. Review the information and instructions in Chapter 1.

❏ **Habit #2 Eating Frequency**
Following is your daily protein requirement. Divide your meals evenly throughout the day, consuming approximately 15 grams of protein with each meal, whether it is real food, a meal-replacement shake or a nutrition bar.

Daily Protein Requirement: _____ grams per day
Daily Eating Frequency: _____ meals per day

If the number of meals required per day proves to be too many for your lifestyle, then you may double up at one or more meals by consuming up to 30 grams of protein, 40 grams of complex carbohydrates, and 12-14 grams of healthy oils per meal. Never eat less than 5 meals that contain 15 grams of protein each, in order to maintain a minimum of 800 calories per day.

Balanced Meal Replacements (MR)

❏ 1 MR Shake/Day   ❏ 2 MR Shakes/Day   ❏ 3 MR Shakes/Day   ❏ 4 MR Shakes/Day

Other:_____
Review the information and instructions in Chapter 2.

❏ **Habit #3 Regular Exercise**
Regular exercise along with proper diet will increase your vitality and slow down the aging process.

❏ **Exercise Plan #1- Low Fit (16-Week Plan)**
*Actual*Age™ score is 10 years or more above your chronological age. Four-week aerobics only program for the low fit. Then move to Plan #2. Follow the instructions for this plan in Chapter 3.

❏ **Exercise Plan #2- Moderately Fit (12-Week Plan)**
*Actual*Age™ score is one to nine years or more above your chronological age. Twelve-week aerobic, strength and flexibility program for the moderately fit. Then move to Plan #3. Follow the instructions for this plan in Chapter 3.

❏ **Exercise Plan #3- Maintaining Fitness (Plan for Life!)**
*Actual*Age™ score equals your chronological age or below. You either measured this way initially or successfully reduced your *Actual*Age™ score by following the 12 or 16-week plans. Either way, Plan #3 is a nutritionally sound, lifestyle-enhanced program that includes aerobic, strength and flexibility maintenance programs to use for life to prevent returning to a low or moderately fit condition. Follow the instructions for this plan in Chapter 3.

❏ **Your Heart Rate Zone (Found in Chapter 3)**
220 Minus Your Age=Your Maximum Heart Rate (MHR)

220 minus _____(age) = _____ (MHR)
❏ Exercise Plan # 1 = MHR multiplied by .50 percent
_____ (MHR) X 0.5 = _____ Beats per Minute (BPM)

❏ Exercise Plan # 2 = MHR multiplied by .60 percent
_____ (MHR) X 0.6 = _____ Beats per Minute (BPM)

❏ Exercise Plan # 3 = MHR multiplied by .70 percent
_____ (MHR) X 0.7 = _____ Beats per Minute (BPM)

❏ **Habit #4 Stimulants** - Gradually reduce your use of stimulants. The benefits can be more energy, increased concentration, more productivity, better sleep and an improved state of well-being. Review the information and instructions in Chapter 4.

Gradually reduce the following stimulants: ❏ Tobacco ❏ Alcohol ❏ Coffee
❏ Tea ❏ Soda ❏ Other_____

❏ **Habit #5 Stress Management** - For optimum health, regular stress management keeps insulin and other hormones balanced. Review the information and instructions in Chapter 5. Consider implementing one or more of the following:
❏ 20-minute walk in nature ❏ Outside deep breathing ❏ Feet up rest breaks ❏ Meditation
❏ Relaxing music break
❏ Other_____

❏ **Habit #6 Supplements** - High quality supplements can help you achieve and maintain proper body composition, slow the aging process and ensure improved health and vitality.

❏ Adhere to supplement recommendations listed on your Personalized Nutrition Prescription

❏ Other/Notes:_____
_____

❏ **Habit #7 Hormone Balance** - This is the ultimate goal of the Healthy Aging Program: when all the Habits are practiced in harmony, enormous health benefits will result. You will feel better, look better and add years to your life and life to your years!
Notes:_____
_____

HOW TO USE YOUR PERSONAL PROGRAM LOG

This log was created so you can easily track daily activities, monitor your progress and achieve success with the Healthy Aging Program. You need to photocopy the master weekly log sheet that follows and keep the completed log sheets in a binder for regular review.

The amount of information you write will probably vary over time. You may go through phases where you want to track every aspect of your program; at other times, you may simply write, "Worked out today."

Even if you record minimal information, it's a good idea to write something every day, and that includes days you don't exercise. This way, when you look back, you'll be able to distinguish between days you rested and days you lacked discipline to follow through. You'll have more clues as to how much the program is truly working for you.

Here is a look at the various sections of the program log, along with sample ways of recording your daily activities. Eventually, you may create a personal way of recording the results that better suits your lifestyle.

Week No:_____
Start each week with the number that represents how many weeks you have been introduced to the program. Even if you take a few weeks off, try to record the correct week. If too much time has elapsed, feel free to begin again at week one.

Date:_____(Month)_____(Day)_____(Year)_____
Be sure to date each week. When keeping the completed log sheets in your binder, keep them in order by the date.

HABIT #1 BALANCED EATING / HABIT #2 EATING FREQUENCY

In this section you can record the number of prescribed balanced meals/snacks you are required to eat each day, and the number of actual balanced meals/snacks you consumed. Refer to the "Personal Program Recommendations" page in this book, which details how much protein you should consume daily and by how many meals you should divide it. Keep in mind that each meal, regardless if it is a meal-replacement shake, nutrition bar or a real food meal, should contain approximately 15 grams of protein and the corresponding percentages of carbohydrates and healthy oils.

Remember, a balanced meal is a meal that has all three of the major macronutrients present: carbohydrates, fats and protein. Each meal should consist of 15 grams of protein, 20 grams of complex carbohydrates and 6-7 grams of healthy oils. You might write:

Number prescribed per day:_____5_____ / Number consumed:_____5_____

HABIT #3 EXERCISE

CARDIO TRAINING
In this section you can record the three different exercise activities, your times and any distance you covered. There's also room to make additional notes, such as how you felt after your workout. For example, if you exercised on the stair climber for 15 minutes at level 5 and then jogged on the treadmill for 15 minutes at 6.0 mph, you might write:

Cardio Training	Time/Distance	Notes
Stair climber	15-min/Level 5	Felt strong
Treadmill	15-min/6.0 mph	Good sweat

If one day you are too tired to stair climb but decide instead to take a yoga class, you could write:

Cardio Training	Time/Distance	Notes
Yoga class	45 minutes	Too tired to run

STRETCHING/FLEXIBILITY TRAINING
In this section, you can record any type of flexibility exercises you conducted. Keep in mind that stretching should not be used as a warm-up exercise. Always stretch after you have warmed up your muscles with at least 5-10 minutes of cardio training. You might write:

Stretching	Time/Type	Notes
Butterfly stretch	15 minutes/lower back	Back feels stronger

STRENGTH TRAINING

In this section you can record your strength-training activities, including how much weight you lifted and the number of sets and repetitions you performed. It's especially helpful to write down the names of the exercises. Writing down "chest fly" will reinforce the idea that the exercise strengthens your chest muscles. If you completed three sets of 10 reps using 45 pounds on the chest fly machine, you could write:

Strength Training	Wt.	Sets	Reps	Notes
Chest Fly	45	3	10	Next time add 5 lbs.

Let's say you perform three sets of machine shoulder press. In the first set you did 15 reps with 50 pounds; the second, 12 reps with 70 pounds; and the third, 10 reps with 90 pounds, you might write:

Strength Training	Wt.	Sets	Reps	Notes
Shoulder Press	50/70/90	3	15/12/10	Strong

If you did three sets of 20 abdominal sit-ups, you might write:

Strength Training	Wt.	Sets	Reps	Notes
Sit-ups	-----	3	20	No back pain

HABIT #4 STIMULANTS

In this section you can record the number and quantity of stimulants consumed. Don't judge yourself if you continue to use these items. Just be aware of your habits and strive to reduce and eventually eliminate your stimulant use. As you better implement the first three habits, you will experience a decrease in cravings for many types of stimulants. You might write:

Stimulants consumed today:
(Coffee/Tea, Soda, Alcohol, Tobacco, Sweets)

Stimulant	Quantity	Notes
Coffee	3 cups	Can't seem to quit
Soda	1 can	Down from 5/day

HABIT #5 STRESS

In this section, you can record the type and length of stress management technique that you are using to reduce stress in your life. Stress reduction is critical to reversing insulin resistance and reducing or preventing Syndrome X. You might write:

Stress management techniques:

Type	How Long	Notes
Walk in nature	20 minutes	Relaxing

HABIT #6 SUPPLEMENTS

In this section, you can record if you are taking any therapeutic foods, meal replacements, and/or supplements that are prescribed for you on a daily basis.

Prescribed supplements taken: (X)Yes ( )No   Notes: Need more Vitamin C

NOTES

In this section you can track specific things like how much water you drank or how many times you became upset in the course of the day. To see how your eating habits affect your exercise performance, you might want to record what you eat before you workout. Over the course of a few weeks, look for any patterns and things to change or continue. This section can be used to record anything that might later be beneficial to continue improving.

WEEKLY WRAP-UP

Here's your chance to look back at the week you just completed. Recording how much you accomplished in one week can give you motivation and direction as you begin the next. By recording if you met or exceeded the goals you set for that week, it will help keep you focused. If you consistently fall short of your goals, maybe you have set them too high or you need additional support. Make a note if you are having challenges with any of the 7 Habits and, in your opinion, if your challenges are due to a lack of knowledge on how and why you need to implement them, or a lack of discipline.

HEALTHY AGING - PERSONAL PROGRAM LOG

Week No:_____(Month)_____(Day)_____(Year)_____

HABIT #1 BALANCED EATING & HABIT #2 EATING FREQUENCY

A balanced meal is a meal that has all three of the major macronutrients present: carbohydrates, fats and protein. Each meal should consist of 15 grams of protein, 20 grams of complex carbohydrates and 6-7 grams of healthy oils.

Number prescribed per day:_____ / Number consumed:_____

HABIT #3 EXERCISE

❏ Plan #1   ❏ Plan #2   ❏ Plan #3

Cardio Training	Time/Distance	Notes
_____	_____	_____
_____	_____	_____
_____	_____	_____

Stretching/FlexibilityTraining	Time/Type	Notes
_____	_____	_____

Strength Training	Wt.	Sets	Reps	Notes
_____	____	____	____	_____
_____	____	____	____	_____
_____	____	____	____	_____
_____	____	____	____	_____
_____	____	____	____	_____
_____	____	____	____	_____
_____	____	____	____	_____
_____	____	____	____	_____
_____	____	____	____	_____

HABIT #4 STIMULANTS

Stimulants consumed today: (Coffee/Tea, Soda, Alcohol, Tobacco, Sweets)

Stimulant	Quantity	Notes
_____	_____	_____
_____	_____	_____
_____	_____	_____

HABIT #5 STRESS

Stress management techniques:

Type	How Long	Notes
_____	_____	_____
_____	_____	_____

HABIT #6 SUPPLEMENTS

Prescribed supplements taken:

( )Yes ( )No   Notes_____

REFERENCES

American College of Sports Medicine, 2nd ed., ACSM Fitness Book, Creative Printing, Hong Kong, pp. 2-13, 1998.

Bland, J. S, Benum, S. H., Genetic Nutritioneering, Keats. Lincolnwood, Illinois pp.104-121, 1999.

Carroll, P.B. and R.C. Eastman. "Insulin Resistance: Diagnosis and Treatment." The Endocrinologist 1.2 (March 1991): 89-97

Collier, G. R. and Sinclar, A. J., "Role of N-6 and N-3 Fatty Acids in the Dietary Treatment of Metabolic Disorders." Annuls of the New York Academy of Sciences. 683 (14 June 1993) 323-30.

Coulston, Ann M., George C. Lui, and Gerald M. Reaven, "Plasma Glucose, Insulin and Lipid Responses to High-Carbohydrate, Low-Fat Diets in Normal Humans." Metabolism 32.1 (1983): 52-56

DeFranzo, Ralph, A. and Eleuterio Ferrannini. "Insulin Resistance: A Multifaceted Syndrome Responsible for NIDDM, Obesity, Hypertension, Dyslipidemia, and Atherosclerotic Cardiovascular Disease." Diabetes Care 14.3 (March 1991): 173-94.

Evans, W. and Rosenberg, I. H, Biomarkers, Simon & Schuster, New York, NY, pp. 1-21, 104-197, 1992.

Facchini, F. Chen, Y.-D. I. And Reaven, G.M. (1994) Light-to-moderate alcohol intake is associated with enhanced insulin sensitivity. Diabetes Care 17:115-119.

Fackelmann, Kathy A. "Hidden Heart Hazards: Do High Blood Insulin Levels Foretell Heart Disease?" Science News 136 (16 Sept. 1989): 184-86.

Hjermann, I., et al. "Effect of Diet and Smoking Intervention on the Incidence of Coronary Artery Disease." Lancet (12 Dec. 1981): 1303-10.

Hoffman, R. L, Intelligent Medicine, Fireside, New York, N. Y., pp. 383-433.

Karam, John H. "Type II Diabetes and Syndrome X: Pathogenesis and Glycemic Management." Endocrinology and Metabolism Clinics of North America 21.2 (June 1992): 329-50.

McArdle, W. D., Katch, F. I., Katch, V. L., Sports & Exercise Nutrition, Lippincott Williams & Wilkins, Baltimore, Maryland, 1999.

Moller, David E and Jeffrey S. Flier. "Insulin Resistance-Mechanisms, Syndromes, and Implications." NEJM 325.13 (26 Sept. 1991): 938-48.

Parillo, M., Coulston, A. Hollenbeck, C., and Reaven, G. M., (1988) Effect of a low fat diet on carbohydrate metabolism in patients with hypertension. Hypertension 11:244-248.

Reaven, G. M., Syndrome X, Simon & Schuster, New York, N.Y, pp. 64-93., 120-131, 2000.

Shen, S.-W., Reaven, G. M., and Farquhar, J. W. (1970) Comparison on impedance to insulin-mediated glucose uptake in normal and diabetic subjects. J. Clin. Invest. 49:2151-2160

Shils, Maurice E., James A. Olson, and Moshe Shike., eds. Modern Nutrition and Health and Disease. 8th ed. Vols. 1, 2. Philadelphia: Lea & Febiger, 1993.

Walden Health Resources, Emotions, Overeating, and the Brain. California: Walden Health Resources, 1993.

Notes:

Notes: